Healthy Eating for Life
for Women

PHYSICIANS COMMITTEE FOR
RESPONSIBLE MEDICINE

John Wiley & Sons, Inc.

This book is printed on acid-free paper. ∞

Menus and recipes by Jennifer Raymond

Published by John Wiley & Sons, Inc., New York
Published simultaneously in Canada

Design and production by Navta Associates, Inc.

This publication is designed to provide accurate and authoritative information in regard to the subject matter covered. It is sold with the understanding that the publisher is not engaged in rendering professional services. If professional advice or other expert assistance is required, the services of a competent professional person should be sought.

Library of Congress Cataloging-in-Publication Data

Healthy eating for life for women / Physicians Committee for Responsible Medicine.
     p. cm.
     Includes index.
     ISBN 0-471-43596-1 (pbk. (alk. : paper)
     1. Women—Nutrition. 2. Women—Health and hygiene. 3. Women—Diseases—Nutritional aspects. 4. Diet therapy. I. Physicians Committee for Responsible Medicine.

RA778 .H44385   2001
613.2'082—dc21   2001046892

Printed in the United States of America

10 9 8 7 6 5 4 3 2 1

Physicians Committee for
Responsible Medicine Expert Nutrition Panel

Healthy Eating for Life
for Women

Neal D. Barnard, M.D.

Patricia Bertron, R.D.

Suzanne Havala, M.S., R.D., L.D.N., F.A.D.A.

Jennifer Keller, R.D.

Gabrielle Turner-McGrievy, M.S., R.D.

Martin Root, Ph.D.

Amy Joy Lanou, Ph.D.

Vesanto Melina, M.S., R.D.

with Kristine Kieswer

Contents

Part II: Making It Work for You

Part III: Lifelong Health

List of Recipes

Foreword

As you open this book, you are opening a door to the very best of health, longevity, and fitness. Much of what you are about to read will be surprising. But you will never look back. Until now, to battle headaches, arthritis, or menstrual cramps, many women have needed fistfuls of over-the-counter remedies. Menopause has meant taking hormones for the rest of your life. Preventing cancer has meant yearly mammograms and precious little else. These approaches are certainly useful. But they are also expensive; riddled with side effects; and, far too often, simply inadequate.

Fortunately, we can now add new, and much more effective, approaches. Through a simple change in your diet, headaches can become things of the past. Menopausal symptoms may never even start. And we can gain new power over the most common and problematic forms of cancer. Everything from improving fertility to erasing the signs of aging to managing osteoporosis, arthritis, and urinary tract infections has been subjected to new methods of research and can now be dealt with more easily than ever. The answer, more often than not, lies in nourishing your body in new and healthy ways.

A few years ago, at the Physicians Committee for Responsible Medicine, working in cooperation with Georgetown University, we began a research study using diet changes to help women with PMS and menstrual pains. Some of our research volunteers had been nearly disabled by pain for a day or two every month, and they were understandably anxious for anything that might help. Many gained remarkable relief (as you'll read in chapter 3). But to me one of the most striking events in this project occurred when one of the new research volunteers arrived at our offices. She wanted to let the team know that if this study had been simply testing another new drug, she would never have volunteered. She—like millions of other women—was tired of treating every medical symptom with pills. She wanted a healthier and more natural way to deal with these problems.

For a great many conditions, we have found them. In this volume we will take a little time to understand how our bodies work and how common health problems arise. Then we will look in detail at how diet and lifestyle adjustments can help. When you are ready to jump in, you will find menus and recipes that put these principles to work. They are easy and delicious and, in fact, are the most pleasurable prescription you will ever fill. But their proof comes in how you feel.

I wish you the best of success and the very best of health.

Neal D. Barnard, M.D.

President, Physicians Committee
for Responsible Medicine

PART I

Essentials

1

Ageproofing
from the Inside

Women know. Skin care—and the business of maintaining a youthful appearance—is a massive industry and is growing each day. Every inch of you, from the delicate skin around your eyes to the heels of your feet, has been analyzed, scrutinized, and studied by scientists in search of better ways to smooth lines, erase imperfections, and brighten complexions. In recent years we've seen alpha and beta hydroxy acids—the new "miracle" cures—added to nearly every brand of over-the-counter skincare product on the shelves. Even mild chemical facial peels are now as quick and painless as a lunch-hour manicure.

The never-ending challenge to alter our appearance has been around forever. Cleopatra lined her eyes with dark kohl crayons. In the 1970s we found a way to bronze our skin with bottles of "sunless tanning" lotion. And today, major facelift surgeries are an everyday affair. It's anyone's guess what tomorrow will bring, but one thing is for certain: This army of researchers, testers, and marketers in a multibillion-dollar industry produces cosmetic changes that are only skin deep. They alter only the thinnest surface of your biology. Scalpels and lasers can temporarily transform our contours, but they can't get to the root of the aging process. Does anyone know what makes those lines creep up around our eyes or why our skin becomes discolored over time? And why do these changes come so fast and furiously for some and much more slowly for others?

What if, long before you'd heard about collagen injections or dermabrasion, you discovered more about *how people age?* If you could "see" what's really going on under your skin's surface, you would be able to strengthen your beauty and vitality from the inside out—repairing, rebuilding, and even preventing the signs of wear and tear from showing up too soon. You could see what causes weight to come on so insidiously, why veins break into unsightly tattoos, and why our bones weaken as we slump into old age. You would take into your own hands a new measure of control.

If you were able to look deep inside the cells of your body, you would see how they vary greatly in size and shape, and how their unique design allows each one to carry out a specific job. Muscle cells allow you to move as they contract and relax. Nerve cells transmit messages. Liver cells eliminate toxins and regulate body chemistry. Red blood cells transport oxygen in and carbon dioxide out. Pancreas cells make and replace hormones. It's a complex, ever-changing universe. Despite its particular task, however, each cell is constructed according to the same basic pattern. Underneath a protective membrane lies a jellylike substance called cytoplasm, which houses the cell's nucleus and all of your chromosomes, each composed of the DNA blueprint that makes you who you are. As hormones, fuel, and nutrients move in and out of the porous cell membrane, all the vital chemical reactions that build and maintain your body take place.

A look inside this intricate world would show you just how fragile your cells are and, more important, how nearly everything you do affects their functioning. You would see how they are assaulted by pollutants you breathe in; how they are defended by certain vitamins and minerals; how they stand up to cigarette smoke and alcohol; and, most important, why some cells deteriorate and others thrive, maintaining their youthful robustness.

What does this have to do with how you look? Understanding what makes a cell flourish gives you the power to make it happen, and your body is more receptive than you probably think. Your eyes, your cheeks, your neck—every part of your body—show the care you've taken to hold the aging process at arm's length.

Gather Your Defenses

Luckily, your body is extremely efficient at defending its precious resources—as long as it has the right ammunition. The area in need of the most focused protection is your cell membrane—the scaffolding material that gives each of your cells the strength to stand tall and strong. When even one molecule in a cell membrane is damaged, a chain reaction can take place, killing the entire cell. As one cell after another dies, wrinkles and other signs of aging are inevitable. Cells with the best chance of surviving the ravages of time are the ones sufficiently packed with special protective nutrients. Found plentifully in vegetables, fruits, grains (bread, pasta, cereal, rice, oats, and corn), and legumes (beans, peas, and lentils), these nutrients pack a mighty punch. As we'll see, some of their natural biochemical defenses actually wedge themselves into protective positions inside your cell membranes, while others unfurl to guard the bloodstream. All of them are strengthened by certain foods you can easily bring into your routine.

Know Your Enemy

Your main adversary in the aging game is the free radical, the molecular piranha that takes bites out of your cells, eventually destroying them. You can't see free radicals—only the damage they leave behind. But as you start to visualize how they operate, you'll learn to protect yourself against their harmful effects. Their modus operandi is this: Free radicals first arrive in your body as benevolent, life-giving oxygen molecules (the ordinary oxygen that keeps each cell alive), but some of these molecules get damaged during various chemical reactions. As you might imagine, oxygen is used in thousands of reactions within your body—building new cells, burning fuel for energy, and endless others, so it is easy for these molecules to be altered in the process. They take on extra electrons or develop

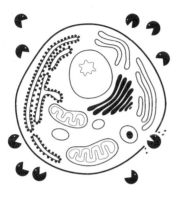

Free-radicals attack a cell membrane, eventually destroying it.

unstable electron orbits of their own. As free radicals, the potential of these unstable oxygen molecules to wreak havoc is enormous. In a lightning-quick fraction of a second, they can demolish any other molecules that get in their way, including your DNA.

This never-ending process destroys minuscule amounts of your body over time, much like crashing waves hitting rocks along a coastline. Whether your body holds up like granite or crumbles like clay depends greatly on what materials you have used in your own cellular construction.

Major Cell Protectors

A certain amount of free radical damage is just a natural part of being alive. When you breathe, when you sleep, and when you eat, free radicals are trying to age you. But you've got an army of nutritional allies on your side. The next time you're thinking of giving yourself a makeover, you may want to start at the grocery store. Each microscopic cell that makes you who you are needs constant nourishment. Here are four cell-protecting powerhouses that will repel free radicals and make your skin, hair, eyes, and whole body thrive.

Selenium. Robust enzymes stand guard over your cell membranes, neutralizing free radicals and stopping destructive chain reactions that have already begun. One of these enzymes requires a special nutrient called selenium to operate properly. Found abundantly in grains, it's easy to get the recommended 50 to 200 micrograms of selenium each day—unless you're skipping the whole grains your body needs. Selenium exists naturally in soil and passes into the roots of grains and vegetables, nourishing the plant as it grows and protecting your body after you eat it.

Notice the word *whole* grains. Four slices of whole wheat bread hold nearly 50 micrograms of selenium. If you choose white bread instead, you'll cut that figure nearly in half, to a mere 28 micrograms. As grains are refined to produce white flour, the mineral-rich outer fiber coating is discarded, along with the selenium that was ready to protect you. So whole grain products are not just more satisfying; they really are much better for you.

Vitamin E. Found in the natural oils of beans, vegetables, fruits, and nuts, as well as in the grains of wheat in your bread, vitamin E is a potent antioxidant that nestles within your cell membranes,

TOP FOODS FOR VITAMIN E (IN MILLIGRAMS)

Almonds (1 oz, dried)	6.7
Avocado (1 medium)	2.3
Brazil nuts (1 oz, dried)	2.1
Broccoli (1 cup*)	1.0
Brown rice (1 cup*)	4.0
Brussels sprouts (1 cup*)	1.3
Chickpeas (1 cup*)	5.1
Corn kernels (1 cup*)	9.3
Mango (1 medium)	2.3
Navy beans (1 cup*)	4.1
Soybeans (1 cup*)	35.0
Spaghetti (1 cup*)	1.0
Spinach, raw (1 cup)	1.7
Sweet potato (1 medium*)	5.9
Wheat germ (1 oz, toasted)	4.0

*Figures refer to cooked servings.

Sources: J. A. T. Pennington. *Bowes and Church's Food Values of Portions Commonly Used,* 17th ed. (Philadelphia: J. B. Lippincott, 1998); and P. J. McLaughlin and J. L. Weihrauch, "Vitamin E Content of Foods," *Journal of the American Dietetic Association* 75 (1979): 647–665.

lying in wait until free radicals come along to threaten it. Instead of attacking your delicate cells, free radicals end up attacking vitamin E. Like swords hitting sturdy shields, the assault is severe, but the damage is minimal. With all of the positive publicity vitamin E has received in recent years, some people have gotten carried away by taking very high doses of it in supplement form. The truth is, you'll get all you need by eating a nice variety of the foods listed in the table on page 7. What's more, vitamin E actually recycles itself. With a little help from your body's supply of vitamin C, it defends your cells over and over again.

Carotenoids. Think carrots, sweet potatoes, pumpkins, and other orange vegetables. Add them to your diet and you'll gain yet another measure of defense against free-radical damage from beta-carotene—the best-known member of the carotenoid family—and its six hundred or so cousins. Delivered to your bloodstream and then to your cells, beta-carotene cloaks them in a protective layer that helps them live longer. Like vitamin E, beta-carotene takes up its post within the cell membrane, repelling invading free radicals.

TOP FOODS FOR BETA-CAROTENE (IN MILLIGRAMS)

Broccoli (1 cup*)	1.3
Butternut squash (1 cup*)	8.6
Carrot (1 medium)	12.0
Collards (1 cup*)	2.5
Kale (1 cup*)	5.8
Mustard greens (1 cup*)	2.5
Pumpkin (1 cup*)	1.6
Spinach (1 cup*)	8.8
Spring onions (½ cup)	1.5
Sweet potato (1 medium*)	15.0
Swiss chard (1 cup*)	3.3

*Figures refer to cooked servings.

Source: J. A. T. Pennington. *Bowes and Church's Food Values of Portions Commonly Used,* 17th ed. (Philadelphia: J. B. Lippincott, 1998).

While carotenoids are particularly concentrated in orange vegetables, they are also found in green and yellow vegetables.

There is a cousin of beta-carotene you should get to know, named lycopene. It has an odd name, but you already know it very well. It provides the red color in a tomato, just as beta-carotene gives its orange color to a carrot or a sweet potato. Slice open a watermelon. Guess where that bright red color comes from? Lycopene may not be as famous as beta-carotene, but it is actually one of the most plentiful carotenoids in your body. It powerfully neutralizes free radicals and has gained popularity among cancer researchers for dramatically cutting cancer risk.

Take a fresh look at the produce aisle. You'll spot nature's palette that has beta-carotene here, lycopene there—not for looks, but for providing strong protection throughout a plant's growing process. When you bring these foods into your diet, their protection enters your skin and all your other body tissues.

The beauty of a diet rich in grains, vegetables, fruits, and legumes is that it provides your body with a rich supply of nutrients for knocking out free radicals and countless other pollutants—without spending a fortune on supplements or thinking in terms of "milligrams" or "recommended daily allowances." Whole, natural foods supply a generous bounty of potent vitamins, minerals, and other protectors for vitality and wellness. Think of Mother Nature as the original Avon lady. When it comes to your healthy good looks, she delivers like no one else can.

Vitamin C. When you drink your morning glass of orange juice, you may think only of its cold-fighting power, but there's a lot more to vitamin C than that. Not only does vitamin C work as a powerful antiaging nutrient, making the collagen that strengthens muscles, bones, and skin, it also helps regulate our moods and psychological functions.

All day long, and even at night as you sleep, free radicals form in your bloodstream. Vitamin C is your blood's number one bodyguard and night watchman, eradicating free radicals with ease. It moves in and out of your cells, joints, brain, spinal cord, and even into your eyes to seek out and destroy free radicals. Eating vitamin C–rich foods such as broccoli, Brussels sprouts, grapefruit, strawberries, and, of course, oranges and other citrus fruits, will send free radicals

TOP FOODS FOR VITAMIN C (IN MILLIGRAMS)

Broccoli (1 cup*)	98
Black currants (½ cup)	101
Brussels sprouts (1 cup*)	96
Cantaloupe (1 cup)	68
Cauliflower (1 cup*)	68
Grapefruit (1 medium)	94
Guava (1 medium)	165
Kale (1 cup*)	54
Orange (1 medium)	80
Orange juice (1 cup)	124
Papaya (1 medium)	188
Pineapple chunks (1 cup)	24
Spinach (1 cup)	16
Strawberries (1 cup)	85
Sweet potato (1 medium*)	28

*Figures refer to cooked servings.

Source: J. A. T. Pennington. *Bowes and Church's Food Values of Portions Commonly Used,* 17th ed. (Philadelphia: J. B. Lippincott, 1998).

and their aging effects packing. Without vegetables and fruits in your diet each day, your defenses will be down.

By now you might feel as if you have to be a chemist to understand all these cell-protecting compounds, but it's actually easier than you think. When you bring home brightly colored vegetables and fruits, along with whole grain breads and cereals, their vitamin E, beta-carotene, lycopene, and selenium automatically enter your cell membranes, while their vitamin C goes to work patrolling your bloodstream. They will defend you against free radicals, slowing down the toll of time.

Healthy Skin and Hair

Now we are starting to see how our outward appearance is truly a reflection of our inner workings, so it's not hard to imagine how our food choices can affect the vibrancy of our hair and the suppleness of our skin. Time alone is not the indicator of how well we age. In fact, the main causes of wrinkles and discoloration of the skin have nothing to do with time. The culprits in skin damage are ultraviolet rays and, not surprisingly, free radicals. But once again, protection is right at our fingertips, not farther than a bottle of sunscreen or any number of cell-nourishing foods.

No one is ever happy to hear that those glowing, rosy cheeks we get from a day in the sun are actually signs of skin damage, but unfortunately it's true. Anytime your skin darkens, it means your epidermis (outermost layer) is trying hard to protect your dermis (innermost layer) from the harmful effects of the sun's ultraviolet rays. The dermis contains collagen protein strands and elastic fibers that give your skin resiliency and strength. When these strands and fibers are damaged and weakened, skin begins to sag. It's something we all wish we had heard more about in our teenage years—not that we would have been likely to listen.

When sunlight hits your skin, 90 to 95 percent of it is absorbed. Your epidermis compensates for this invasion by shedding its outer layer to reveal fresh skin. And, as our skin "tans," another change is going on: Skin cells and protein fibers deep inside your skin are also being damaged. And you need not stand in direct sunlight for this to occur. Ultraviolet rays bounce off of the ground and diffuse through the sky before they reach you.

Protect Your Skin—Outside

Regardless of your age, it's never too late to stop sun damage in its tracks. Many facial moisturizers and foundations now have an added sun-protection factor (SPF). This is good news because most people don't think about sun protection unless they plan to spend a day at the pool or the beach. But daily sun exposures from strolling to lunch, sitting in the park, or walking your dog really add up over time. Used daily, an SPF of 15 or higher will help prevent wrinkles, depigmentation, and little brown "age spots" as well as precancerous skin changes. It's a good idea to stay out of the midday sun; take advantage of the protection that clothing, sunglasses, and hats provide; and avoid tanning beds, as the ultraviolet A rays they emit penetrate the skin deeply.

This is not to say that you should avoid the sun entirely, because the sun provides benefits as well. Fifteen minutes of sunlight each day on any part of your body is necessary for normal vitamin D metabolism, and the sun has an uncanny ability to elevate our moods. Like many other things, it's good in small doses, but can turn harmful in excess.

Protect Your Skin—Inside

Dark-skinned people have better built-in protection from ultraviolet rays compared to light-skinned people, simply because darker skin produces more melanin. But, no matter what shade of skin we're born with, we can all improve our body's own SPF internally, with the foods we choose.

As we saw earlier, eating carrots, sweet potatoes, and other orange or green vegetables sends a dose of protective beta-carotene to our cells and bloodstream. This phytochemical is our best internal defender against excess ultraviolet radiation. Some plants contain so much beta-carotene that they are able to withstand endless hours in direct sunlight, neutralizing free radicals. When you eat beta-carotene-rich foods, you are packing these same powerful nutrients into your cell membranes, defending yourself from excess sun exposure and free-radical damage. You've likely heard about the effects of excessive beta-carotene consumption—people turning themselves a pale shade of orange. While this is a harmless (and temporary) side effect of overdoing a good thing, the invisible antioxidant and immune-boosting actions taking place inside you are quite effective.

Having said that, you will still want to be cautious in the sun. Even the world's best diet is no match for hours of baking under summer rays. Use the internal protection of a beta-carotene-rich diet along with external protection, not in place of it.

Healthy Eyes

Remember when your parents said you would keep your good eyesight if only you'd finish your carrots? Well, there's truth to what probably seemed like a bit of parental bribery. A diet that includes carrots, or any other vegetables and fruits, sends beta-carotene, vitamin C, vitamin E, and many other antioxidants into your eyes, neutralizing harmful free radicals stimulated by the daily sunlight exposure most of us receive. The carotenoids in orange, yellow, and green vegetables help discourage macular degeneration, a loss of function of the retina found in older adults. Avoiding tobacco and excess dietary iron (as we will see shortly), and, of course, wearing sunglasses all help keep your eyes healthy.

You may never have heard of macular degeneration, but sooner or later you'll hear more about it than you ever wanted. It is the most common major assault on vision that occurs as the years go by. You'll learn of a friend or a relative who is gradually losing sight, and the deterioration can continue to total blindness. It is worth taking a minute to understand how certain foods protect the tender, paper-thin retina in your eyes, because these foods do exactly the same thing for your skin and every other part of your body.

As intense, focused light hits your retina, sparking the production of free radicals, carotenoids are front and center to knock them out. Researchers from the Massachusetts Eye and Ear Infirmary and many other medical centers around the world found that people who get the most carotenoids in their diet had a 43 percent lower risk of macular degeneration compared to people who get the least. Macular degeneration is the leading cause of blindness in people over sixty-five. The most powerful sources of carotenoids are spinach and collard greens.

Of course, what you *don't* eat counts here, too. Steer clear of fatty foods, especially animal fats, to naturally hinder free-radical production, which can slow down blood flow in the eye's tiny arteries. As a matter of fact, the same people who succumb to heart attacks are also at high risk for macular degeneration, suggesting that the same fatty diets may be partly to blame. Researchers writing in the journal *Ophthalmic Epidemiology* found that people with macular degeneration had precisely the same risk factors as heart disease patients: a high-fat diet, smoking habits, hypertension, and diabetes. It appears that damage to delicate blood vessels is the root of the trouble.

Here is the take-home lesson: The daily beating your eyes take in the line of fire of focused light, minute after minute, is not so different from what happens to your forehead, your temples, your neck, and every other part of your body. Sunlight and other elements can easily assault you, and if you do not protect yourself with the right foods, they will age you at a quickened pace. All parts of your body need the same protection.

Drinking milk, which has been indicted in a number of troubling health concerns, also can cause eye problems for some. As milk products are digested, they produce a simple sugar called galactose, which can enter the lens of the eye. Infants who are unable to break the sugar apart develop cataracts, a cloudiness in the lens that impairs vision, within the first year of life. Population studies have shown that adults who live in regions where dairy products are commonly consumed have much higher rates of cataracts than those where dairy products are rarely consumed. Because the troublemaker here is the milk's sugar and not the fat, using skim variations offers no protection.

Iron—Too Much of a Good Thing?

There is a surprising side to iron—a treacherous and harmful side that accelerates the aging process by encouraging free-radical production. Iron is a very unstable metal. An iron pan can rust rather quickly. In your body, iron oxidizes even faster, producing free radicals along the way. Although iron is an essential nutrient, it is dangerous in excess. But you'd never know it by the way it has been marketed, especially to women. Not so long ago, advertisements promoting iron supplements as a cure for fatigue and all kinds of other difficulties were everywhere. These ads are gone now, and with good reason. In reality, there is rarely a need to add extra iron to your diet and, given the way most of us eat, iron *overload* is more of a cause for concern than iron deficiency.

A trace of iron in your blood (in the form of hemoglobin within your red blood cells) allows it to carry oxygen—a function necessary for life. However, your body carefully sequesters any surplus, storing it in special molecular containers called ferritin. Each one can hold up to forty-five hundred iron atoms inside its protein shell, safeguarding you from the iron overload that would result if iron were left free to roam in the bloodstream. Ferritin also protects you from iron deficiency that may arise from bleeding or dietary inadequacy, by serving as an emergency reserve.

Why does your body work so hard to balance its iron supply? Because it knows that free-floating iron is dangerous. You can safely hold 100 to 300 milligrams of iron in your body, but when levels reach 800 milligrams or so—the amount present in more than half of us—iron hastens the destruction of your body's tissues. A chain reaction in a cell membrane can destroy it, and the results are wrinkles and aging in other body tissues.

Iron overload can accelerate aging in other ways, too. It can make its presence felt in the form of fatigue, arthritis, weakness, impotence, diabetes, shortness of breath, loss of menstrual periods, and neurological problems. Most important, excess iron is a major contributor to heart attacks. The only way to know for sure if your iron level is safe is to have your blood tested at a clinic or your doctor's office. The tests outlined here are much more accurate than standard hemoglobin or hematocrit blood tests, which are not sufficient.

How to Check Your Iron Level

Your doctor or clinic can run the following tests. In some states, commercial laboratories will run these tests without a doctor's request. A physician should always interpret the results.

- serum ferritin (normal values are 12 to 200 mcg/l)
- serum iron
- total iron-binding capacity (TIBC)

Serum iron should be checked after an overnight fast. The serum iron measurement is divided by the TIBC. The result should be 16 to 50 percent for women and 16 to 62 percent for men. Results above these norms indicate excess iron. Results below these norms indicate too little iron. If the result suggests iron deficiency, your doctor may request an additional test called a red cell protoporhyrin test for confirmation. A result higher than 70 mcg/dl of red blood cells suggests insufficient iron. To diagnose iron deficiency, at least two of these three values (serum ferritin, serum iron/TBC, or red cell protoporhyrin) should be abnormal.

Plant Iron vs. Animal Iron

The dangers of iron overload are easily avoided when you fill your plate with plant foods. Iron is abundant in beans and lentils and also is found in vegetables and grains. If your body is low in iron, the vitamin C from fruits and vegetables will bolster its absorption. Even premenopausal women who lose blood with each menstrual period can easily replenish their iron requirements with a rather modest amount of beans and vegetables. In fact, premenopausal women are the group most likely to have proper iron balance, while men and postmenopausal women are prone to iron buildup, forcing their bodies to make more and more ferritin to quickly store it away.

When you boil, steam, or stir-fry your vegetables, you increase their usable iron even further. No matter how many iron-rich vegetables you eat, your body can easily handle it, absorbing the amount of iron your body needs. It sounds like a perfect system and it nearly is, until you add red meat, poultry, and fish to your diet. That's when iron overload begins.

Meats contain a form of iron called heme iron, which comes from the hemoglobin in an animal's red blood cells and other tissues. Quite different from plant iron, it simply doesn't comply with your body's own iron-regulating system. Regardless of how much iron you already have stored in your body, heme iron barges through your intestinal wall and into your bloodstream, adding to free-radical activity and damaging your cells. In this case, taking vitamin C supplements can make matters worse by further increasing iron absorption.

It is very common for people in Western countries to have excess iron, especially as they reach middle age. If you are one of them, you'll want to stop the influx of more iron by cutting out meat, poultry, and fish, and relying on vegetables, fruits, grains, and legumes to keep your nutrients in better balance. Exercise also reduces iron levels through the excretion of sweat and urine. Believe it or not, you can quickly reduce excess iron levels by giving blood. As your kind donation benefits those in need, you'll safely reduce the number of harmful free radicals in your body—two reasons to feel good. Those who are unable to donate blood due to infectious illness, low blood pressure, or other reasons should seek the assistance of their physician.

People with normal or low iron stores will benefit from adding vitamin C–rich fruits and vegetables to their diet without risk of overdoing it. A true iron deficiency, found by taking the tests above, doesn't mean that you should add meat to your diet. Vegetables and beans are the healthiest iron sources available. Your doctor also may prescribe supplements for temporary use. Also since dairy products inhibit iron absorption, avoiding them generally helps your body naturally regulate its iron balance.

Oils

Ever since fats and oils made the top of the "hazardous to your heart" list, there has been talk of which oils are worst and which are best. The short answer is that all oils, including vegetable and fish oils, can be detrimental to your health in one way or another, whether they are lurking in your stir-fry or are baked into your foods. While there are data to suggest that some people can safely add olive oil to foods, the healthiest dishes are generally made without any added oil.

Tropical oils—palm, coconut, and palm kernel—provide a hefty dose of saturated fat. And, just like animal fats, they stimulate your liver to produce more cholesterol. When checking food labels, be wary of oils that are fully or partially hydrogenated. This indicates that the oil has been chemically saturated (solidified) to increase its shelf life; but it also increases your cholesterol. Liquid oils such as peanut, sunflower, and corn oils are better from the standpoint of cholesterol, but they cause problems of their own. If you've left liquid oils unrefrigerated for a time, you know they eventually turn rancid. These same molecular changes take place inside your body, creating free radicals and paving the way for the damage they cause.

Whether the oils you use are solid or liquid, some part of your body will take a beating when they are in your foods. Liquid vegetable oils are much better than animal fats and tropical oils, but you would do your heart and skin a tremendous advantage by learning to prepare foods with little or no oil. You may be pleasantly surprised to rediscover the zesty flavors of vegetables and other foods so often drowned in heavy sauces and creamy dressings. The recipes we will look at later in this book rerelease the true flavor of fresh foods.

The Trouble with Alcohol

While some people say "a little wine is good for you," evidence is clear that more than a little can do real damage. You can certainly see this in the signs of alcoholism: Skin begins to sag, and eyes look tired and worn out, not to mention the injury an alcohol-soaked liver endures. But you don't have to drink excessively for your cells to suffer. When you drink, alcohol molecules enter your body, rearranging themselves into various forms of harmful free radicals and encouraging more oxygen molecules to do the same.

That's right—alcohol causes free radicals to form. While your inhibitions go down and your pain tolerance goes up as you drink, alcohol-produced free radicals harm the stomach, heart, and other organs. And, as we will see later, alcohol also increases your risk for breast cancer.

Confusion concerning the pros and cons of moderate alcohol consumption still exists. Wine lovers rejoiced when news reports suggested that drinking red wine protects the heart. After all, heart disease rates appeared to be lower in France, a country famous for its high-fat delicacies. A sobering investigation by the World Health Organization put these statistics in a very different light. It turned out that French death certificates had recorded many heart attacks simply as "sudden death," while other nations listed them as cardiac deaths. Using the same record-keeping methods, the French have about the same heart disease rates as other Western nations.

And since you've just learned about the hazards of excess iron, it's wise to note that red wine is brimming with it. Combined with its alcohol content, which makes iron more absorbable, you've got a double whammy in your wineglass. All the while, it is depleting the antioxidants you were so mindful to ingest.

You may have found some of the information in this chapter surprising. Physicians, nutritionists, and dietitians who specialize in preventive medicine have made great strides in recent years to uncover the keys to remaining youthful and vigorous. Fortunately, for the rest of us, their discoveries are quite simple to implement. We've covered important principles. Now let's see how to put them to work.

2

Making Sense
of Nutrition

In the previous chapter we looked at how foods can help minimize the signs of aging. But let's back up and think, not in terms of aging, but *living,* because that's what you plan on doing for as long as possible, in the healthiest possible body. Every part of you is constantly changing. In fact, your liver, skin, and blood cells are completely replaced several times a year. What you ate for breakfast contributes nutrients to every cell in your body, determining how healthy you'll be, and even affecting the way you feel right now. Just imagine what a week's or a month's worth of nutrients can do. A decade's worth of mediocre meals will create one scenario, while a decade's worth of nutrient-packed meals will certainly create quite another—not just in the arteries of your heart, but also on the surface of your skin, in the glow of your eyes, and in the spring in your step.

The protection that certain foods provide simply cannot be duplicated in a pill or a superficial cosmetic treatment. Their nutrient makeup is as complex as each cell in your body. And each cell knows just how to maximize the benefits of every vibrant red pepper and bright yellow squash you eat. Multiply that by the more than a hundred million cells that make you who you are and you've got a body fueled by good nutrition and fit for *living!*

New Four Food Groups

At first, good nutrition may seem daunting and tricky. An easy place to begin is by eating at least three servings of vegetables and three servings of fruit each day. Orange vegetables such as carrots and sweet potatoes; dark, leafy vegetables such as broccoli, spinach, kale, and mustard greens; and an assortment of fruits contain the antioxidants your cells need to block out free-radical damage. Eat your favorites, but don't hesitate to try new kinds, as the recipes at the back of the book will help you do.

Begin your lunch or dinner with a salad of raw vegetables such as spinach, cucumbers, zucchini, sweet peppers, and tomatoes, with a sprinkle of chickpeas. Packages of washed, cut, and ready-to-eat vegetables, found in many grocery stores, are great time-savers. Selecting a variety of plant foods will give each antioxidant—and there are many specialized kinds—the opportunity to defend you to the fullest extent.

Experiment with new dishes centered around grains, beans, and lentils. These foods will invigorate your cells with new strength. But we're getting ahead of ourselves. Let's trace out the basics of a healthy diet, and translate nutritional science into breakfast, lunch, and dinner.

In 1991, physicians and scientists from the United States and England introduced the concept of the New Four Food Groups as a way to put recent nutritional discoveries to work. Much improved from the old food groups popularized in the 1950s and simpler than the Food Guide Pyramid, the new plan was rich in good nutrition while containing no animal fat or cholesterol at all. Although it was hotly controversial when it was first proposed, it has withstood the test of time and remains the most scientifically sound nutritional plan yet devised.

Here are the New Four Food Groups, with details on how to use them:

Whole Grain Group

Whole grains are dietary staples in countries with the greatest longevity and best overall health. Beyond whole grain breads, which most of us love, you can enjoy old-fashioned oatmeal and other breakfast cereals, corn, and a variety of colorful pasta—the Asian invention, perfected in Italy, that comes in every shape and size. Exquisite rice dishes such as curries, pilafs, and Latin American specialties differ in taste and texture.

What nutritional treasures are found in grains? Lots of fiber, complex carbohydrates, important vitamins, and a healthy amount of protein—not too much or too little. They fit easily under the 10 percent fat limit used in Dr. Dean Ornish's study of reversal of heart disease (which we will explore further in chapter 8) and contain no cholesterol.

Vegetable Group

Vegetables have become all too unfamiliar on American dinner plates, and you certainly won't find many on fast-food menus. All the while, daily news reports confirm findings of yet another naturally occurring compound found in vegetables that helps fight cancer or boost immunity. Broccoli and other greens are loaded with calcium, carbohydrates, fiber, and vitamins. Vegetables tend to be very low in fat and, like all plant foods, contain no cholesterol. A diet without a nice range of daily vegetables is dangerously low in essential nutrients.

Fruit Group

Fruits range from apples, bananas, cherries, oranges, and other familiar foods to kiwis from New Zealand, cherimoya from Ecuador and Peru, and carambola (starfruit) from southern China. They are rich in vitamins, carbohydrates, and soluble fiber—powerful artillery against heart disease, cancer, and weight problems. Fruit is great for breakfast, dessert, or as a major part of any meal.

Legume Group

The term refers to beans, lentils, and peas. Americans are familiar with navy beans and a few other varieties, but many cultures have made skillful use of the full range of legumes. Lentils make delicious soups or curries. Chickpeas are pureed with garlic and scallions to become Middle Eastern hummus (a dip for pita bread) or formed into a spicy falafel patty. Black beans, gently flavored with tomatoes, peppers, and onions, are a savory staple of Latin American cuisine. And, of course, bean burritos covered in fresh salsa are an easy Mexican treat. Legumes are rich in protein, carbohydrates, fiber, and minerals, while they are low in fat, have no cholesterol, and are a good source of omega-3 fatty acids.

Eating should be a pleasurable experience, not one filled with guilt and anxiety about unhealthy foods you may be eating. The New Four Food Groups allow that to happen with ease. Proportion guidelines are presented below. They are, of course, quite broad and can safely be adjusted according to your size and daily activities. An athlete in training would require more calories than the average woman, but as long as they are both consuming the majority of foods from whole grain sources, plenty of vegetables and

Daily Servings

- Grains: Five or more servings (a serving = 1 ounce of dry cereal, ½ cup of hot cereal, 1 slice of bread, ½ cup of cooked rice)
- Vegetables: Three or more servings (a serving = 1 cup of raw or ½ cup of cooked vegetables)
- Fruits: Three or more servings (a serving = 1 medium piece of fruit or ½ cup of fruit juice)
- Legumes: Two to three servings (a serving = ½ cup of cooked beans, 8 fluid ounces of soy milk)

Be sure to include a source of vitamin B_{12} from a multivitamin or fortified cereals, rice milk, or soy milk. Look for the words "cobalamin" or "cyanocobalamin" on supplement labels, which are chemical names for vitamin B_{12}. Our daily requirement for B_{12} is just 1 mcg, an amount that can easily be reached even when you include it every few days.

fruits, and two or three servings of legumes, they are eating well. On a healthy diet, your appetite is a good indicator of when to eat and when to put down the fork. The New Four Food Groups are so low in fat, you'll be able to eat until you are satisfied. And there is no need to worry about eating cereal in the morning and vegetables in the evening. Eat according to your cravings. If cereal with soy milk and fruit is your idea of a great late-night snack, enjoy.

Foods That Didn't Make the Cut

Let's look at what's *not* included in a healthy menu. Chances are you'll find a surprise or two. The new science of nutrition has led a great many people to break some old habits, with wonderful results in the process. Here are the food products we've learned to avoid.

Meat, Poultry, and Fish

Foods have always found their way into women's beauty treatments. Cool cucumbers to reduce puffiness around the eyes. Avocado extracts to comfort upset skin. Almond oil to smooth cuticles. If they do the job, more power to you.

When we think about healing nutrients, we think of foods nourished with the earth's goodness. Chicken and beef don't quite conjure images of refreshment or renewal, do they? Scientists aiming to reverse heart disease or prevent cancer have soured on these products, too, finding they do more harm than good. Most people have gotten the message that too much red meat can spell real trouble for the heart, waistline, and other organs. Unfortunately, many have turned to chicken and fish in their pursuit of better nutrition. These cuts are lighter—*in color*—but your body can hardly tell the difference. Virtually all nutritional authorities now recommend basing your diet not on meat, fish, or poultry, but on grains, vegetables, and fruits, a recommendation strongly echoed by the federal government's U.S. Dietary Guidelines.

Why the tendency to minimize animal products? Because chicken, fish, and virtually all other animal products contain a hefty dose of cholesterol, fat, and animal protein, while they leave your body wanting for fiber, vitamins, and complex carbohydrates.

Oftentimes the heaviness of a meat-centered meal leaves little room for what your body really needs—a rich variety of plant foods. And given the current state of agricultural and environmental affairs, animal products often harbor even more unpleasant surprises than we bargained for.

Here's a rundown of why you'll want to skip the meat group:

Fat and cholesterol. Meats contain a surprising amount of fat. Even the leanest beef gets nearly a third (29%, to be exact) of its calories from fat, most of it in the form of artery-clogging saturated fat. All meats contain cholesterol, which is different from fat, and which you can think of as a kind of glue that holds the cell membranes together.

There is no longer any question that the less meat you eat, the better. Research studies that have successfully reversed heart disease use vegetarian diets—that is the only way to eliminate cholesterol.

As health problems caused by meat and other animal products became clear in one research study after another, it was a logical first step to cut back on the foods in question—we surrendered to skim milk, skinned our chicken, and switched to fish. But instead of the dramatic improvements we hoped for, these changes often just lead to a frustrated feeling of deprivation. It's no wonder why. Chicken contains just as much cholesterol as beef, and its fat content is nothing to celebrate either. Even without the skin, chicken is still 20 percent fat and often much more, depending on the variety. Compared to the leanest cuts of beef at 29 percent fat, it's easy to see why a switch from beef to chicken makes minimal differences to our bodies. As we saw earlier, some types of fish have even more cholesterol than red meat.

Heart patients are often placed on the National Cholesterol Education Program Step II Diet to lower their risk for future heart attacks. This involves limiting meat products to six ounces per day, trimming the skin and visible fat, and having egg yolks no more than once per week. Even those who strictly adhere to the diet, carefully counting every last gram of fat, generally see a drop of just 5 to 6 percent in their cholesterol numbers. That's not enough to prevent heart attacks, and it requires a lot of effort for little reward. No one calls their attention to the tremendous amount of fat in animal products compared to rice (1 to 5%), beans (4%), or potatoes (less than 1%) so they will see the real solution as their problem. All foods from plant sources are free of cholesterol, and nearly all are very low in fat, unless it is added in the kitchen.

As with all animal foods, fish gives you a significant dose of fat and cholesterol. They do vary, so you will get 40 milligrams of cholesterol in a 4-ounce piece of tuna and about twice that in rainbow trout. Most surprising is the amount of cholesterol in mobile shellfish such as shrimp and lobster. Ounce for ounce, shrimp have *double* the cholesterol compared to beef.

Although fish and fish oil capsules have been touted for their omega-3 fatty acids as a means for lowering heart disease risk, they encourage the production of free radicals, which you want to minimize for many reasons. When you choose foods from healthier sources, as we will soon explore, you naturally and safely lower your risk for heart disease and other serious illnesses. The omega-3 fatty acids from fish are highly unstable molecules, decomposing quickly and unleashing free radicals in the process. The kind you will find in vegetables, fruits, and beans *reduces* free-radical activity while adding antioxidants. It's a double dose of protection you can get at every meal.

Uninvited Dinner Guests

Chemicals

Fish are hardly swimming in pristine waters: Our waterways are receptacles for sewage systems and pesticide runoff. The National Research Council reports that polychlorinated biphenyls, or PCBs (industrial chemicals used in electrical equipment, hydraulic fluid, and carbonless carbon paper), are found in virtually every site where fish or shellfish have been tested—even in remote spots off Alaska and Hawaii. These contaminants become densely concentrated in fish muscles and then find their way into your body, where they remain for many, many years.

The Food and Drug Administration (FDA) stopped testing fish for mercury in 1998, although previous tests showed potentially unsafe levels of mercury present in tuna, swordfish, and shark. Eating fish tainted with mercury has been shown to contribute to Parkinson's disease, a condition of abnormal muscle control, as well as depression, irritability, and other psychiatric symptoms. One large sampling of shellfish found that of 145 sites tested, every single one contained mercury. As fish consumption is, by far, the greatest route of exposure, avoiding fish is the only way to eliminate this risk. When you skip the fish, you cut your exposure in half.

In March 2001, the FDA released a warning advising all pregnant women, women of childbearing age, breastfeeding women, and children to avoid predatory fish such as shark, swordfish, and mackerel because of their high levels of methyl mercury.

Ciguatera, a cousin of *Pfiesteria,* is found in reef fish such as grouper, jack, barracuda, and snapper. The toxin causes numbness, tingling, nausea, vomiting, headache, weakness, irregular heartbeat, and sometimes death in those who contract it. Notoriously hard to diagnose, its symptoms have been found to linger for more than ten years in some people.

There are a million or more ciguatera poisonings annually around the world, with cases reported in Florida, Vermont, and Texas. Because cooking does not destroy the toxin and it is not visible in fish who carry it, health reports advise us not to eat the head, eggs, or guts of predatory fish. On second thought, why not order the pasta, salad, and vegetable soup?

Chicken, our most popular "white meat," looks harmless enough dressed up in the drive-thru special of the week. But zesty new sauces and an expensive marketing campaign can't disguise its shortcomings. Chicken is by no means light, low-fat, or remotely healthy.

You wouldn't dream of taking daily antibiotics, and certainly not veterinary medicines, in your quest for good health, but if you are choosing chicken salads and chicken sandwiches for lunch most days, you're doing just that. To keep up with demand, farms today operate like high-tech factories. Thousands of chickens are confined in small cages piled one on top of the other. Excrement and other forms of bacteria fall through the cages and are spread in every direction. Stressed by these unnatural conditions, chickens often peck at one another, causing serious injury. To protect profits, birds are routinely debeaked, which obviously raises ethical concerns as well. You can't tell by looking, but the neatly wrapped chicken breasts that you see in the grocery store may still harbor antibiotics and other medications used to compensate for these troublesome conditions. Vegetables and fruits are not injected with hormones. And even when they are treated with pesticides, they cannot concentrate them the way animals do in their body fat. With a growing market of health-conscious shoppers, many large health food stores are able to offer an immense selection of produce, much of which is organic (not treated with pesticides). Even mainstream supermarket chains are expanding their selection of fresh produce so you should have no trouble finding that perfect purple eggplant, a bundle of broccolini, and many new additions. Unlike PCBs, which are slow to leave the body, chemicals from medicated feed and various veterinary compounds are easily eliminated when we get away from meat. In a comparison with the general population, women who adopt a vegetarian diet have 98 percent lower levels of several pesticides and other chemicals in their bodies.

Bacteria

One of every three chickens in the supermarket cooler has live salmonella bacteria growing inside its plastic packaging. And it is easy for chickens to pass the disease through their ovaries and into their eggs. Cooking eggs "sunny side up" doesn't destroy the bacteria. And don't forget about the raw eggs in popular foods such as Caesar dressing, hollandaise sauce, eggnog, mousse, and homemade ice cream. Salmonella and other microorganisms kill approximately nine thousand Americans each year and, in less serious cases, cause vomiting, diarrhea, abdominal pain, and fever often mistaken for the flu. In infants, the elderly, and people with compromised immune systems, the infection can be fatal. Unfortunately, there are eight other major foodborne pathogens, including the well-known *E. coli* and *campylobacter,* commonly found in animal products (and most chicken packages) posing a continual threat to those who consume them. In case you were wondering, the USDA's "seal of approval" ensures only that the product is free of "visible" signs of disease.

Carcinogens

If you thought the trouble with chicken could be cooked away, there's more bad news. Chicken produces dangerous heterocyclic amines (HCAs) when it is heated. Produced from creatine, amino acids, and sugar in the chicken muscle, HCAs also are found in tobacco smoke, and are fifteen times more concentrated in grilled chicken than in beef. The combination of fat, animal protein, and carcinogens found in cooked chicken also creates troubling risks for colon cancer. At the same time, poultry, like all meat, lacks the fiber needed to cleanse the digestive tract of excess hormones and cholesterol. Each bite of beef, chicken, and fish that you eat displaces vegetables, whole grains, and legumes—the real dynamos that give your metabolism and immune system a boost.

Got (Problems with) Milk?

Dairy products are a big part of culinary traditions in America, Western Europe, and many other countries. Whatever the dish, someone is smothering it with cheese. Fast-food eateries could probably sell a cardboard sandwich if they covered it in three kinds of cheese. But when your goal is to change the role that foods play in your life and to start using them to your best advantage, it's time to take a good, hard look at dairy.

Let's begin with milk. Modern dairy farming presents much of the same contamination issues as chicken farming. Cows graze on pesticide-soaked lands and, since the legalization of bovine growth hormone (BGH) in 1993, farmers have been using it to produce enormous quantities of milk. As a result, cows often develop mastitis, a painful udder infection that must be treated with antibiotics. Again, these chemicals can end up in your carton of milk, adding to the problem of antibiotic resistance and other health risks. Twenty different antibiotics and thirty-three other drugs are legal for use in dairy cows.

Organic milk products are available in some grocery stores; however, pollutants are not the only reason why dairy products do not belong in an optimal diet. Every slice of cheese you add and every glass of milk you drink, other than skim varieties, burdens your body with fat and cholesterol. Given the very high fat content of whole cow's milk (49% of its calories are from nothing but fat), it's clear that nature never intended adult humans to consume it at all. What's nourishing to a calf has caused a multitude of problems for human beings.

Risks associated with the consumption of dairy products include insulin-dependent diabetes, prostate cancer, osteoporosis (see chapter 10), allergies that can cause respiratory distress, canker sores, skin conditions, cataracts, asthma, and, surprisingly enough, fertility problems in women. Babies often suffer from a digestive irritation called colic. It has long been known that eliminating cow's milk formula often solves the problem. A study in the journal *Pediatrics* found that women using dairy products pass milk antibodies along to their babies when they breastfeed, increasing the chance of causing colic.

As we have seen, iron deficiency in Western countries is uncommon. But add milk products and this can change. Low in iron to begin with, milk often displaces iron-rich foods in the diet. In infants it can cause irritation and loss of blood from the intestinal tract, which over time reduces the body's iron stores. Even combining a healthy food such as broccoli with cheese or milk reduces its usable iron by about half. While adults often have problems with iron overload, as we saw in the previous chapter, iron deficiency in children is risky, and dairy products often are contributors.

Milk causes unnecessary discomfort for people who are lactose-intolerant. Even though 95 percent of Asian Americans, 74 percent of Native Americans, and 70 percent of African Americans cannot digest dairy's lactose sugar, milk products have been pushed in the U.S. Dietary Guidelines for all Americans. All babies have lactase enzymes, which allow them to digest milk. But for many, these enzymes disappear after childhood, so milk drinking causes cramping, diarrhea, and nausea. About 85 percent of Caucasians tolerate milk sugar, but only because of a genetic mutation passed down from distant ancestors. About 75 percent of people worldwide do not. Apparently nature has ensured that mother's milk—in all mammals—contains ideal nutrients for infants. After this stage of life, milk is no longer needed—especially milk from another species—and a new set of nutrients is required.

Perhaps the most troubling side of milk relates to a compound called insulin-like growth factor, or IGF-I. There are small traces of IGF-I in your bloodstream normally, and it has many biological functions, from encouraging cells to grow, to storing nutrients. But IGF-I also is a powerful stimulus for cancer cell growth. Researchers believe that in even slight excess, it may be linked to higher risk of prostate cancer in men and breast cancer in women. Here is where milk comes in. Researchers have found that drinking milk regularly can boost the amount of IGF-I in your blood by about 10 percent, precisely the opposite of what you want to happen. Perhaps this explains why several studies have found higher cancer rates in countries where milk drinking is especially popular.

A Diet for Optimal Wellness

America's love affair with high-fat, low-fiber foods has taken its toll. More than half of Americans are overweight. Our insides are being attacked by heart disease, diabetes, cancer, osteoporosis, and other painful and costly diseases. Our outsides are expanding, sagging, and deteriorating far too early in life. And many people are desperately trying to find their way back to health.

The easiest way to pack life-enhancing foods into your day is to begin with a whole new idea of "what's for dinner." The New Four Food Groups turn old ideas about nutrition upside down. Why worry about how much your chicken breast weighs when you can feel satisfied eating regular portions of fresh, flavorful foods? The New Four Food Groups put vegetables, grains, fruits, and legumes back in the heart of your recipes, where they can nurture your cells, knock out harmful free radicals, and keep extra weight away.

Making a Healthy Breakfast, Lunch, and Dinner

What does healthy eating look and taste like? For breakfast you won't want to go near bacon or eggs, which are fattening up far too many people. So how about a big bowl of old-fashioned oatmeal topped with cinnamon and raisins, along with half a cantaloupe, and some hearty whole grain toast? If you really have to have the taste of bacon or sausage for a while, new vegetarian versions are tasty enough to fool the most skeptical, food-dissecting child at your breakfast table.

Healthy lunch at the office is as easy as heating a bowl of soup. Lentil, black bean, minestrone, and split pea are good choices.

Browse the health food aisle of any major supermarket for vegan selections full of vegetables, beans, noodles, and delicate spices instead of chicken or beef broth. Add a ready-made salad (pre-cleaned and precut) with your favorite fresh veggies (carrots, cauliflower, tomatoes, cucumbers, onions, celery, etc.) and a whole grain roll. Perhaps a veggieburger or sweet potato, which are easily cooked in the microwave. Flavored hummus with pita bread triangles are a nice variation. And, of course, a fresh fruit cup is always a smart choice.

When you start to rethink dinner, you'll surely want to experiment with new foods and recipes. For starters, however, you can easily cook up some whole-wheat spaghetti with chunky tomato sauce, a quick veggie and rice stir-fry with steamed tofu, or a cheese-free pizza loaded with your favorite toppings.

As for proportions, let about a third of your plate be covered with whole grains such as brown rice or whole grain pasta. Then bring in the vegetables as generously as you can, filling about half of the plate, and have more than one kind—say, carrots with spinach, or sweet potatoes with broccoli. The remainder of your plate should contain a legume: lentils, beans, or peas.

By now you may be wondering, Will I get enough protein? Will I get calcium? The answer to both these questions is a resounding yes. Let's look at getting complete nutrition.

Key Nutrients—Where They Are and How They Work

Protein

Busy women are all in search of more energy and stamina. You may have wondered if you're getting enough protein. After all, advertisements have loudly portrayed meat, especially beef, as the superior protein source. Today we have a much better understanding of how much protein we need for good health and where to find the best sources. Protein is needed to build and repair body structures, from tiny blood cells to major organs. Even so, excess protein doesn't equal better health. There are serious risks associated with eating too much.

More complicated than most carbohydrates or fats, protein molecules are made up of long, twisted strands of amino acids that contain nitrogen. From just twenty amino acids, your body makes endless numbers of proteins to build and regulate your body's muscles, skin, bones, cells, and many other life functions.

A more than adequate supply of protein for a normal, active adult can easily be found in a varied diet of vegetables, fruits, grains, and beans. If you had bacon and eggs with cereal and milk this morning, you have overdosed on protein before noontime. Trying to purify your bloodstream of the nitrogen it leaves behind in your body, your liver and kidneys must work extra hard.

In recent years, high-protein diets have come into vogue. Like all fads, such diets are recycled through bookstores intermittently over the years. Each time they resurface, people desperate to lose weight buy into the idea, often to their serious detriment. There is no need to be one of them. High-protein diets emphasize meat and eggs to the near-total elimination of grains and other carbohydrate-rich foods. If they succeed at temporarily shedding pounds, it is largely from the diet's diuretic effect, in addition to the fact that these diets are old-fashioned, low-cal diets. They drain your body's precious water supply and deprive you of important nutrients, and, over the long run, this is quite dangerous. Besides the doses of fat and cholesterol these meat-heavy diets add, they rob your body of essential minerals, especially calcium.

When researchers feed animal protein to volunteers and test their urine, they find it loaded with calcium. Here's why: When protein is digested, its component amino acids come apart and pass into the blood, making the blood slightly acidic. However, the body is extremely finicky about how acidic the blood gets, because even a tiny change can derange body chemistry. In the process of neutralizing the acidity, calcium is pulled from bones and ends up being lost in the urine. It's as simple as that: As animal protein goes in, calcium goes out. The more animal protein you eat, the greater your risk for osteoporosis.

If you were thinking you could just replace all that lost calcium with a glass of milk, think again. Milk does contain calcium, but its load of protein increases your body's calcium losses at the same time. Even high-dose calcium supplements will not counteract the effects of a lifelong, high-protein diet in preventing bone loss.

Attaining proper calcium balance is a matter not just of getting more and more calcium but also of eating a balanced diet that includes green vegetables, beans, and fortified juices, and avoiding animal protein. And go for a walk. The importance of regular exercise in maintaining a strong, healthy posture cannot be overemphasized.

Just look down the street and you'll probably spot dozens of restaurants serving meat, cheese, or eggs (or all three) in every breakfast, lunch, and dinner item on the menu. It's no surprise that Americans consume more than twice the amount of protein necessary for good health. Eating a variety of foods from the New Four Food Groups will provide you with all the protein your body needs, without increasing your risk for heart, bone, and kidney diseases.

Superior Calcium Sources

Recent advertising campaigns have promoted the notion that everyone desperately needs more calcium and that our failure to drink enough milk has led to osteoporosis and bone breaks. This idea has been marketed so aggressively it is probably hard to imagine there is quite another side to milk. However, scientific studies have produced some surprising results.

First, milk does not protect against osteoporosis. The Harvard Nurses' Health Study followed 77,761 women aged 34 to 59 over a twelve-year period and found that those who drank three or more glasses of milk per day had no reduction in the risk of hip or arm fractures, compared to those who drank little or no milk. In fact, milk drinkers' fracture rates were slightly *higher.* Among those who got the most calcium from dairy sources, hip fracture rates were nearly double those of women who had little or no dairy in their diets. A large Australian study found exactly the same thing.

Many other calcium researchers have found that countries with the highest calcium intakes actually have higher, not lower, rates of osteoporosis. The reason may lie in other concomitant dietary characteristics. Where calcium intakes are highest, large dairy industries exist, producing not only large quantities of milk, cheese, yogurt, and butter, but also meat from dairy cattle whose milk production has declined. Where meat consumption is greatest, osteoporosis rates are high. As we saw earlier, the animal protein from beef, chicken, fish, eggs, and even dairy products forces calcium out of your body.

A group of Yale researchers looked at hip fracture rates in sixteen different countries, focusing on women over fifty because osteoporosis is particularly aggressive in women after menopause. They found that countries with a high calcium intake happened to be those where Western diets—high in meat and dairy products—were popular. Again, the more meat people ate, the more fractures they had.

A report in the *American Journal of Clinical Nutrition* showed that when research subjects eliminated meat, cheese, and eggs from their diet, they cut their calcium losses in half. How much calcium do you actually need? Unfortunately, scientists haven't finished debating that question. On the one hand, Americans lose a great deal of calcium through their urine, due to the animal protein, sodium, and caffeine they consume, aided and abetted by physical inactivity. So some nutritionists argue for ever-increasing calcium intakes to try to make up for the losses, on the order of 1,000 milligrams per day, or even more. On the other hand, researchers have clearly shown that the populations with the strongest bones and lowest fracture rates have fairly modest calcium intakes, and they also tend to avoid animal protein. In China, Japan, and much of the rest of Asia, for example, cheese, milk, and ice cream have never been dietary staples. Calcium comes from vegetables and bean products, and typically meets the World Health Organization's guideline of 400 to 500 milligrams per day.

To keep calcium in your body where it belongs, you'll first want to stay away from animal proteins that drain it from your body, and keep sodium to a minimum, too. It's an aggressive calcium depleter.

Refer to the following chart of calcium-rich plant foods to determine whether you're feeding your bones what they require to stay strong. Osteoporosis prevention is covered extensively in chapter 10.

HEALTHFUL CALCIUM SOURCES (IN MILLIGRAMS)

Black turtle beans (1 cup, boiled)	103
Broccoli (1 cup, boiled)	178
Brussels sprouts (8)	56
Butternut squash (1 cup, boiled)	84
Celery (1 cup, boiled)	54
Chickpeas (1 cup, canned)	78
Collard greens (1 cup, boiled)	14
Cornbread (2-oz piece)	133
English muffin	92
Figs, dried (10)	269
Great Northern beans (1 cup, boiled)	121
Kale (1 cup, boiled)	94
Kidney beans (1 cup, boiled)	50
Lentils (1 cup, boiled)	37
Lima beans (1 cup, boiled)	52
Navel orange (1 medium)	56
Navy beans (1 cup, boiled)	128
Onions (1 cup, boiled)	58
Orange juice (calcium-fortified, 1 cup)	300*
Pancake mix (¼ cup, 3 pancakes)	140
Pinto beans (1 cup, boiled)	82
Raisins (⅔ cup)	53
Soybeans (1 cup, boiled)	175
Sweet potato (1 cup, boiled)	70
Tofu (½ cup)	258
Vegetarian baked beans (1 cup)	128
Wax beans (1 cup, canned)	174
Wheat flour, calcium enriched (1 cup)	238
White beans (1 cup, boiled)	161

*package information

Source: J. A. T. Pennington. *Bowes and Church's Food Values of Portions Commonly Used,* 17th ed. (Philadelphia: J. B. Lippincott, 1998).

Carbohydrates Make a Comeback

Sometimes it seems as if there is a conspiracy against your good health. While protein is getting undeserved praise in fad diet books, healthy carbohydrates have been banished from the dinner plates of misguided dieters everywhere. So many people are missing out on pasta, rice, lentils, potatoes, bread, and even vegetables for fear that they will turn to fat.

The truth is, carbohydrates are not fattening. They are not even especially high in calories. A gram of carbohydrate from potatoes, bread, or pasta has only four calories, while a gram of fat from chicken, beef, or other sources has nine. In fact, as long as carbohydrates are not loaded down with fatty sauces, oils, or butter, they can promote aggressive weight loss. The next time you are choosing items from the food bar or supermarket, consider this: Six ounces of black beans contains 150 calories, while six ounces of skinless chicken breast has 280 calories. Complex carbohydrates are naturally low in calories. Even better, they *cannot add directly to your body fat.* In fact, if you were to really overdo it on carbohydrates, your body has a tough time turning them into fat. The conversion of a carbohydrate molecule into a fat molecule is complex and energy-consuming, using a full 23 percent of calories in the process. In contrast, beef or chicken fat can easily add to the fat on your body, and only 3 percent of their calories are used in the conversion.

Best of all, carbohydrates increase your metabolism—your basic calorie-burning speed—for a few hours after each meal. These calories are lost as body heat, not stored as fat. Here's the skinny: Researchers at the University of Rochester asked a group of young men to drink a special carbohydrate solution, and then measured their metabolic rates. Blood tests showed that their calorie-burning speed increased and remained elevated for more than 2½ hours. All the while, the subjects did no exercise, but rested comfortably in bed. Carbohydrates are like personal trainers for your cells. Each time you choose rice, pasta, or potatoes—cooked healthily—you're giving your body an internal, fat-burning workout. Employ them each day—in place of meat and dairy products—and you will see the results. The New Four Food Groups allow you to choose generous amounts of vegetables, grains, legumes, and fruits so you'll never have to think in terms of what you *can't* have again.

Iron: Not Too Much, Not Too Little

Iron is essential for red blood cells to carry oxygen to your body tissues. Previously, we saw the importance of being careful about iron to minimize free-radical production. The New Four Food Groups provides healthy nonheme iron from plant sources, allowing your body to absorb what it requires while avoiding excesses. By steering clear of burgers and fried chicken you will greatly reduce the fat/iron combination that can easily contribute to free-radical damage.

Zinc

Zinc is important for normal growth and many other body functions. As with iron, it is best to allow foods such as grains, corn, oats, peas, potatoes, spinach, and other plant foods to supply your daily requirements, rather than boosting your zinc level too high with supplements. Excess zinc has been linked to immune system damage and has Alzheimer's researchers paying close attention as well. One study, testing the ability of zinc to improve alertness in Alzheimer's patients, ended abruptly when the supplemented patients quickly began to deteriorate. It is safest to avoid supplements and rely on a well-rounded vegetarian menu.

Aluminum

Unlike iron and zinc, which our bodies require in trace amounts, we need no aluminum at all. Unfortunately, aluminum sneaks in from soda cans, aluminum pans, some brands of antacids, and even many deodorants. Kidney patients on dialysis are often exposed to high levels of aluminum, which can lead to abnormalities in the brain. Aluminum is often found in drinking water and, like other metals, has been implicated as a possible culprit in Alzheimer's disease. Your local health department can tell you more about the quality of your water.

Riboflavin

Also known as vitamin B_2, riboflavin helps make enzymes that are used for many essential body functions. When you are low in this vitamin, you may have skin problems, anemia, or other disorders. You'll get riboflavin by eating asparagus, broccoli, mushrooms, avocados, Brussels sprouts, and peas. Although your intake of riboflavin will be a bit less than if you had eaten animal products, the amount you need, called the Dietary Reference Intake, is actually very low, about 1.3 milligrams per day for men and 1.1 milligrams for women. A study led by Dr. Colin Campbell in the People's Republic of China found average intakes of well under a milligram per day, yet no signs of deficiency were seen.

Vitamin B_{12}

Vitamin B_{12} is an interesting vitamin in that it comes from bacteria. Neither animals nor plants produce it, although plants can be contaminated with it from touching the soil, and animals harbor it, produced by bacteria in their intestines.

The recommended intake for B_{12} is only 2.4 micrograms per day, a minuscule amount. And the body does such a magnificent job of conserving this vitamin that people can go for years on a diet low in B_{12} without developing a deficiency.

Nevertheless, B_{12} is important. It is crucial to cell division and proper nerve functioning. A deficiency, although rare, would indeed be serious and may present symptoms such as anemia and neurological problems such as weakness, tingling in the arms and legs, and a sore tongue. When you choose foods from the New Four Food Groups, you should include a source of B_{12} such as fortified breakfast cereals, soy milk, meat analogues, or Red Star brand (Vegetarian Support Formula) nutritional yeast. A simple multivitamin or B_{12} supplement will do just as well. Look for the word "cobalamin" or "cyanocobalamin," which are chemical names for B_{12}.

Anytime you surf the Internet for health news or listen to a medical report on the evening news, you're likely to hear about new discoveries in how certain nutrients work to protect your cells and organs. Now that you've built your menu from healthy foods, whatever scientists are spotlighting at any given moment will already be in your cabinets or refrigerator in the form of wholesome foods. There's usually no need to run out and buy supplements or overload your diet with the high-profile food of the hour. With a balanced diet of plant foods, you'll cover your wellness bases. Now let's see how foods affect a woman's reproductive cycle and delicate hormonal balance.

PART II

Making It Work for You

3

Diet and the
Menstrual Cycle

Ask any grandparent about their grandchildren and they are likely to mention "how fast they grow up." A young person today will witness more technological and cultural changes before high school graduation than older generations did in an entire lifetime. And, while sweeping technological advances are changing how much of the world communicates, works, and travels, they are also dramatically altering how foods end up on our plates. In North America, meals at home have been replaced by fast food, and snack food is now everywhere. In Asia, similar influences have allowed an influx of burgers, chicken, and hot dogs to replace traditional rice, noodle, and vegetable dishes. Our bodies, and now theirs, have been hard pressed to cope.

The dangers of growing up on fatty, meaty, overprocessed convenience foods are now very clear as heart disease, cancer, diabetes, high blood pressure, and many other illnesses have become epidemics. But there are more subtle changes, too—biological effects of unhealthy diets—that occur surprisingly early in life.

The majority of girls in Western nations reach puberty at about 12½ years of age. Half of African American girls are now showing signs of puberty by age 8. It wasn't always so. World Health Organization records show that in 1850, the average age of menarche (the first menstrual period) was about 17. Over the past 150 years, it has slowly but steadily fallen. The reason for the decline appears to be gradual changes in our diets. Highly refined and processed foods have edged out vegetables and fruits. Meat and dairy products have taken center stage in many meals—even breakfast. Time and again, when various regions of the globe become Westernized, traditional foods made of whole grains, vegetables, and beans are abandoned in favor of cheeseburgers, chicken "strips," and greasy fries. In the process, dietary fat skyrockets and healthy fiber and vitamins are lost. As we will see, these diet changes increase the amount of sex hormones in a child's bloodstream and, with their hormones unnaturally elevated, girls and boys reach puberty earlier in life. Besides the emotional and societal challenges that early sexual maturity brings, it can have lasting effects on our health—especially for women.

Later we will see how the factors that drive early puberty also can lead to a more difficult menopause and even an increased risk for breast cancer. But first let's see how foods affect a woman's basic hormonal cycle.

You may not think about it until the week before your period begins, but the hormones in your body are constantly in flux. Your ovaries make several kinds of estrogens (although for simplicity we will refer to them collectively as *estrogen*) and progesterone, each of these sex hormones playing a unique role in reproductive functions. For North American women, an average menstrual cycle lasts about twenty-eight days. At the beginning of each cycle, estrogen levels slowly rise, causing the lining of the uterus to thicken in preparation for pregnancy. In about two weeks, as estrogen drops, an ovary releases an egg, which passes into the fallopian tube and then into the uterus. Along the way, fertilization can take place. Taking over where estrogen left off, the ovary then starts to manufacture progesterone, the "pregnancy promoter."

The Hormonal Cycle

Progesterone signals the walls of the uterus to fill with blood vessels to nourish a growing baby. If the egg is fertilized, the ovary

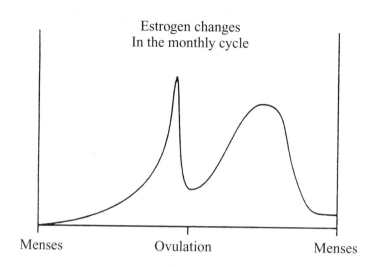

Estrogen changes
In the monthly cycle

Menses   Ovulation   Menses

There is very little estrogen in the bloodstream when a woman's monthly cycle begins. Over the next two weeks, the amount of estrogen rises rapidly, and then suddenly drops around the time of ovulation. Over the next two weeks, estrogen rises and falls again, and then the whole cycle begins anew.

keeps on making progesterone. If not, production is halted and the lining of the uterus is shed (menstruation). These hormones have many other functions, too. Estrogen is responsible for the changes that occur in girls at puberty, and both estrogen and progesterone influence bone strength.

Foods That Calm Hormonal Tides

The foods we eat have a dramatic effect on these hormonal cycles. Foods you may have grown up eating—meats, cheese, eggs—easily drive hormonal levels up. Just as fatty foods make your cholesterol level rise, they do the same to your estrogen level. And, the more fat you have in your diet, the higher these estrogens go. This happens with all kinds of fat whether if comes from meat, dairy products, or from oils used in cooking. So as estrogen levels begin to rise with the start of each menstrual cycle, fatty food causes them to rise more steeply and to reach higher levels in your bloodstream. In the days before your period, estrogen levels finally drop. How far they have to drop depends on how high they were to begin with. On a high-fat diet, the drop from an artificially high level and back down again will be sharper. This "estrogen withdrawal" can cause a variety of problems, from painful periods to difficult menopause. In populations where more traditional, plant-based diets are still regularly consumed, women have lower estrogen levels and longer menstrual cycles—that is, a longer time between each menstrual period. This means they have less exposure to estrogen hormones throughout life and an easier time with many hormone-related changes—simply from dining on hearty breads; rich bean, pea, and lentil dishes; and plenty of vegetables.

The best way for a woman to calm hormonal shifts is to avoid the foods that cause them. Exchanging fatty foods for natural plant foods—more whole grain bread, pasta, and cereal, a variety of vegetables, fruits, and legumes—prevents estrogen levels from entering the danger zone.

The advantage of these foods comes not only from being lower in fat, important as that is. The key ingredient in these foods, as physician Denis Burkitt established in his groundbreaking research, is fiber. Foods from plant sources contain an abundance of natural fiber, which is completely missing from animal sources.

Practicing surgery in Africa for more than twenty years, Burkitt questioned why certain diseases, so common in America and Europe, were rarely seen in less developed nations. His research showed that the dramatically lower rates of colon, rectal, and breast cancer he saw in his patients were partly due to the amount of fiber and lack of fat in their diets. Here's what he found:

After each meal, bile acids in the intestines go to work to absorb fat. Bacteria in the intestines turn some of them into cancer-promoting secondary bile acids. When there is plenty of fiber, less of these acids turn dangerous, while at the same time excess acids are soaked up. Fiber also sweeps away cholesterol. These findings held the promise of dramatically cutting cancer and heart disease rates, and Dr. Burkitt and his colleagues became deservedly famous in the medical community. But it turns out that the very same process works to rid your body of excess estrogens. These estrogens are filtered out of the bloodstream by the liver, passed down through a tiny tube called the bile duct, into the intestinal tract, where fiber carries them away.

In a Dutch study, researchers observed the eating habits of young girls and measured the hormones in their blood. They found that those who consumed more vegetables and grains had lower estrogen levels and reached puberty later in life. The girls who ate more vegetables got about 20 grams of fiber per day, just slightly more than the other group, though it was enough to delay puberty. This means a lower risk of any of the problems caused by excess estrogens, including cancer, in the future. When you consider how much fiber a total vegetarian menu provides—30 to 40 grams per day—you can imagine what it does to smooth out hormonal surges.

Plant foods protect in three powerful ways. First, they drastically reduce the amount of fat in your diet. According to the National Cancer Institute, cutting your fat intake in half will lower your estrogen levels by about 17 percent. Second, the fiber in plant foods naturally helps your body get rid of excess hormones. Third, plant-based diets increase the amount of sex-hormone binding globulin (SHBG) in the blood. These special protein molecules hold on to estrogen and testosterone until they are needed. They keep hormones in check, promoting a more stable menstrual cycle and reducing cancer risk. Studies have shown that, in men, having more SHBG in the blood can mean a less aggressive and domineering personality—not a bad side effect.

The table on the following page compares the amount of fat in a variety of animal products and plant foods. It's easy to cut the fat in your diet simply by switching the *type* of foods you eat, rather than reducing portions.

As you can see, plant foods are usually very low in fat. There are a few exceptions, such as avocados, nuts, olives, seeds, and tofu. They are fine for occasional use, and contain valuable nutrients of their own, but you'll want to keep them to a minimum to maintain a very low-fat diet.

Premenstrual Syndrome—Causes and Cures

If you don't pay close attention, the only connection you may make between hormonal changes and the foods you eat is the candy bar craving that comes during the week before your period. Of course, there is more to premenstrual syndrome (PMS) than food cravings.

FAT IN COMMON FOODS (IN PERCENTAGE OF CALORIES)

PLANT FOODS	FAT	ANIMAL PRODUCTS	FAT
Apple	5	Top loin	40
Banana	5	Top round	29
Peach	2	Halibut	19
Baked beans	4	Chicken (skinless, white)	23
Black beans	4	Roasted chicken	51
Broccoli	8	Short loin	64
Peas	3	Atlantic cod	8
Potato (baked)	1	Salmon	52
Spinach	7	Ground beef ("extra lean")	54
Macaroni	4	Turkey (skinless, white)	18
Brown rice	5	Striped bass	22
White rice	1	Swordfish	30

Source: J. A. T. Pennington. *Bowes and Church's Food Values of Portions Commonly Used,* 17th ed. (Philadelphia: J. B. Lippincott, 1998).

In fact, PMS can encompass many symptoms—up to 150 as recorded by researchers—ranging from mild to debilitating, depending on the individual.

PMS affects approximately 40 percent of women of childbearing age, but has come under serious scientific scrutiny only in the past three decades. The most common symptoms can include breast tenderness, bloating, backache, headache, irritability, nausea, depression, acne, and reduced concentration. Not surprisingly, diet has a lot to do with it. As we have seen, the hormone shifts that lead to PMS can be dramatically affected by how much fat and fiber are in the diet. Cutting the fat reduces hormone shifts, and increasing fiber helps eliminate excess hormones.

Putting vegetarian foods to the test, doctors at the Physicians Committee for Responsible Medicine and Georgetown University conducted a study examining the effect of diet on PMS and menstrual pain. For two months, participants were asked to eat a low-fat vegan diet (containing no animal products) of vegetables, grains, fruits, and legumes, with no restriction on quantity. They also avoided oils, fried foods, nuts, avocados, and olives to create a diet made up of approximately 10 percent fat.

Many participants in the vegan diet group were delighted to find a reduction in both the duration and the intensity of menstrual pain. Many also found relief from the concentration problems, constriction of social and work interactions, and water retention that come along with PMS. Women in this group also lost an average of one pound per week.

How do foods affect menstrual pain? The painful cramping in the uterine muscles comes from prostaglandins, chemicals made from traces of fat stored in cell membranes. The researchers hypothesized that if women reduced their fat consumption, they would in turn decrease their estrogen levels, which would reduce cell growth and prostaglandin production in the uterine lining. The goal was to use foods that even out the hormonal highs and lows many women experience each month. And it worked. For many, the change was so profound that they were reluctant to return to their old eating habits later, even when the researchers asked them to. They had less pain, more energy, and lost weight—and they wanted to stay that way.

Other Factors Affecting PMS

Other aspects of your diet can affect how you feel throughout your menstrual cycle. Let's look at current findings on certain food ingredients, medications, and natural remedies you may not have considered.

Calcium

There is evidence that getting into better calcium balance can ease menstrual pain, especially milder varieties. In one study, calcium carbonate supplements (1,000 mg per day) reduced both menstrual pain and PMS symptoms. A combination of calcium and magnesium also reduced pain and premenstrual water retention while improving mood and concentration.

It is important to remember, however, that attaining ideal calcium balance is not just a matter of adding more calcium, but also keeping the calcium you have. Animal proteins force your kidneys to remove too much calcium from the blood and excrete it in the urine. By keeping animal products out of your diet, you can cut your calcium losses in half. By including green, leafy vegetables, beans, lentils, and other calcium-rich plant foods and fortified orange juice in your diet, you will ensure that you get plenty of calcium and that it stays where it belongs.

You can further reduce your calcium losses by:

- avoiding excess salt and sugar
- limiting coffee to two cups per day
- avoiding tobacco
- exercising regularly
- getting vitamin D from the sun or a multivitamin

It is best to avoid getting calcium from dairy sources because of the significant animal protein and sodium load they provide, which serves to deplete much of the calcium they contribute. And surprisingly enough, only 30 percent of the calcium they contain is readily absorbed in your body. Most vegetables and beans have plenty of low-fat, highly absorbable calcium. Magnesium-rich foods such as soybeans, beet greens, black-eyed peas, and tofu aid calcium absorption even further.

Phytoestrogens

Many vegetarian foods and Asian specialties made from soy such as miso soup, tofu, and tempeh contain weak plant estrogen called phytoestrogens. These natural plant estrogens provide benefits in two important ways. First, they attach to the estrogen receptors on your cells, preventing much of your own estrogen from doing so, therefore preventing unwanted activity on the cell. Less estrogen activity can mean a reduction in menstrual symptoms, as we have seen, and also reduces the odds that cells will turn cancerous, as we will see later in the book.

Interestingly, phytoestrogens have the opposite effect for women after menopause. When your natural estrogen production wanes, plant estrogens may help to bolster it, reducing hot flashes and other menopausal symptoms. In essence, soy foods and vegetarian foods work as a sort of "estrogen regulator" throughout life, helping to make each hormonal change easier.

Caffeine

Caffeinated coffee, teas, and sodas are popular pick-me-up beverages, but they also can aggravate PMS symptoms. Many women who eliminate caffeine from their diets find relief. Trading soda for water also can help reduce bloating and prevent dehydration, which can cause fatigue and mental sluggishness.

Sugar

If you are reaching for sugar-filled candy bars and cookies before each period, these cravings may actually have been triggered by what you have been eating *throughout* your entire cycle. Cravings may be a symptom of "estrogen withdrawal," aggravated by high-fat (estrogen-boosting) foods eaten over the entire month, and controlled by consistently eating nutritious, low-fat foods.

That said, it is important to note that sugar affects different people in different ways. Initially, sugar increases a brain chemical called serotonin, which plays an important role in moods and sleep. The more sugar there is in a meal, the more serotonin your brain will produce. For some, this effect is a pleasurable one. For others, it causes irritability, fatigue, and depression, and very sensitive people can be adversely affected simply by drinking fruit juice regularly. A few days of sugary foods—even juices—can be all it takes to send them into depression.

To test whether sugar is the culprit in premenstrual moodiness, try eliminating all sugars (including natural fruit sugars) from your diet. Researchers have speculated that some people crave sugar to naturally compensate for inadequate levels of serotonin in their brains. But be careful not to confuse the immediate bliss of a sugary snack with long-term well-being. Monitor your moods throughout the day to get a feel for how your body handles sugar.

Unlike simple sugars, complex carbohydrates are made of a long string of sugars that are released gradually after they are eaten. Some, such as beans and green, leafy vegetables, also have plenty of protein and fiber to balance them nutritionally, and they release their natural sugars more gradually than others, such as potatoes and white bread.

Prozac

About 60 percent of women who suffer from mood disturbances each month find relief from selective serotonin-reuptake inhibitors (SSRIs) such as Prozac, Zoloft, or Paxil. The dose used to treat PMS is smaller than that used for depression and is therefore less likely to cause side effects. Several other medications are available when SSRIs do not help.

Vitamin B_6

Vitamin B_6 (pyridoxine) has been shown to reduce pain in some studies by increasing the neurotransmitters that inhibit pain sensations. Vitamin B_6 also has been shown to help combat depression, irritability, and other symptoms in research studies. Spinach and soybeans are high in B vitamins and can help ease symptoms naturally. B vitamins have other useful effects as well, including helping remove estrogens from the liver. A diet low in B vitamins may allow estrogen levels to rise. Look at the following table to see whether you have been including these healthy vitamin B_6 foods in your diet.

Natural Progesterone

We saw how estrogen dominates during the first half of the menstrual cycle and progesterone during the second half. Among other roles, progesterone counteracts the effects of estrogen, preventing too much stimulation of the uterus. However, if your ovary doesn't release an egg—a so-called anovulatory cycle, which is not uncommon in some women—no progesterone is made.

One way to bring back hormonal balance is by using natural progesterone cream. Extracted from yams and soybeans and concentrated in a laboratory, its structure is an exact duplicate of human progesterone. Although synthetic variations do exist, they can cause side effects. A common and convenient brand of transdermal progesterone cream is Pro-Gest, available from Transitions

HEALTHFUL SOURCES OF VITAMIN B$_6$ (IN MILLIGRAMS)

Avocado (1)	0.85
Banana (1)	0.66
Broccoli (1 cup, boiled)	0.22
Brussels sprouts (1 cup, boiled)	0.46
Chickpeas (1 cup, boiled)	0.23
Kidney beans (1 cup, boiled)	0.21
Lima beans (1 cup, boiled)	0.30
Navy beans (1 cup, boiled)	0.30
Pinto beans (1 cup, boiled)	0.27
Potato (1, baked)	0.70
Soybean flour (1 cup)	0.57
Spinach (1 cup, boiled)	0.44
Sweet potato (1 cup, boiled)	0.80
Vegetarian baked beans (1 cup)	0.34

for Health (800-648-8211). It is not recommended for women using oral contraceptives because they are getting progesterone from the pills themselves.

For relief of menstrual pain, a two-ounce jar of progesterone cream is gradually applied to the skin over ten days, using up the jar just before the period is expected to begin. For some, smaller doses are effective. The cream should be applied to thin areas of skin such as the neck, upper chest, abdomen, and insides of the arms and legs, covering as wide an area as possible and varying areas to which it is applied. Allow two to three months to see benefits. Stopping the progesterone on the twenty-sixth day will allow your period to occur normally. If PMS symptoms continue, you may need a higher dose. Use 30 to 40 milligrams per day (about half of a 2-ounce jar per month) from day fifteen through twenty-six, until symptoms diminish. The rationale for a higher dose is that emotional tension is accompanied by the release of the "stress hormone" cortisol, which competes with progesterone for receptors on the cells.

Exercise

Regular aerobic workouts can do wonders for your mind and body. Activity can help shed excess pounds and weight-related problems, reduce fluid retention, and alleviate stress. Exercise also releases endorphins (natural feel-good chemicals) in your brain to lift your spirits and ease mood disturbances.

Essential Fatty Acids

As mentioned earlier, prostaglandins, made from traces of fat in our cells, are among the main causes of menstrual pain and cramps. Reducing dietary fat decreases estrogen levels and prostaglandin production in the uterine lining. But it is not just the amount of fat that matters. It's also the type. When you reduce your dietary fat in a healthy way by eating more beans, peas, lentils, and a variety of vegetables rather than eating "lean" meats, low-fat dairy products, or "reduced fat" snack foods, you'll get a nice helping of omega-3 fatty acids. You also can add ground flaxseeds to your cereal or bake it into your pancakes, muffins, or bread. This type of fat increases your production of helpful prostaglandins, the kind that inhibit inflammation. This often leads to milder menstrual symptoms. You can find omega-3s in a convenient form in flaxseed oil, normally taken as one to three teaspoons per day. And a diet rich in vegetables and beans in place of meat and dairy products will supply traces of these nutrients as well.

There will never be a shortage of medications designed to mask the pain of menstrual symptoms and to counter other symptoms of hormonal changes. Sometimes they are just what you need for temporary relief. But painkillers don't address the cause of the problem. As with so many health concerns, the easiest and best place to begin is with a healthy change to your diet. Better hormonal balance and smoother transitions will likely be found on your dinner plate.

4

Enhancing Fertility

Few women make dietary and lifestyle decisions with their reproductive health in mind. It's usually not until a woman wants to have
a child that she starts learning more about the intricate workings of
her reproductive system. Even then, nutrition rarely enters the pic-
ture. But the time you start planning for a family is a great time to
evaluate your diet. Surprisingly enough, certain foods tend to
enhance fertility, while others may inhibit it. As you improve your
diet to encourage conception, you will also get a measure of protection against other reproductive diseases, including ovarian cancer. And you will likely protect your heart and trim your waistline
at the same time. In fact, the foods you choose during pregnancy
may even affect your child's health far into the future. Of tremendous benefit as well are the habits you will establish with your part-
ner and for your future family. Nurtured in a household where
healthy eating is an enjoyable experience, without anyone dieting or
feeling bad about food, children will be more likely to carry good
eating habits into their adult lives.

Menstrual Cycle Disturbances

As we saw in the previous chapter, a high-fiber, low-fat diet keeps estrogen levels under control and can help ease painful menstrual symptoms. It also can have an effect on the menstrual cycle itself. To have the best chance of conceiving, each intricate reproductive function, including ovulation, must occur properly each month. It's a delicate system. As a new cycle begins, your ovaries make estrogen in ever-increasing amounts to ready the uterus for pregnancy. Two weeks into the cycle, one ovary releases a tiny egg. As the egg descends through the fallopian tube toward the uterus, timing is critical. It has just a few precarious days to unite with a sperm cell and implant on the uterine wall, where, hopefully, it will grow into a healthy baby.

Cycles gone awry may manifest as the absence of menstruation, infrequent menstrual flow, or anovulation, when no egg is released (often occurring with no visible symptoms).

One study from the University of British Columbia comparing ovulatory function between two groups of women—one vegetarian, the other nonvegetarian—found that the vegetarians had fewer ovulatory disturbances. The vegetarians' advantage apparently came from the diet's hormone-taming effect. As we saw in the previous chapter, avoiding animal products and keeping vegetable oils low help you avoid wild swings in the amount of estrogen that courses through your bloodstream, which can easily occur on fattier diets. And vegetables, fruits, beans, and whole grains provide the extra protection of fiber, helping to eliminate excess estrogens.

The benefits of a hormone-balancing diet are seen in better fertility, reduced menstrual symptoms, and most important, in its measure of protection against breast, uterine, and ovarian cancer. The effects are more far-reaching than you might have guessed. As a recent study has shown, a mother's estrogen level during pregnancy can even affect her daughter's risk for developing breast cancer later in life. Researchers from Harvard University and Sweden found a 30 percent increased risk for babies who weighed more than eight pounds at birth—an indicator of estrogen levels in pregnancy.

A Surprising Danger in Dairy Products

As we saw in chapter 2, the majority of people, excluding Caucasians, have trouble digesting dairy products because they do not retain the enzymes for digesting milk sugars after infancy. Even though most Caucasian women—about 85 percent—have the genetic adaptation that allows them to eat dairy products without experiencing intestinal discomfort, it doesn't necessarily mean that they are protected from the long-term negative effects elsewhere inside the body. Dairy can turn the ovaries into a silent battleground.

Ongoing research by Daniel Cramer, M.D., at Harvard Medical School has shown how dairy products can affect the ovaries: When you eat or drink dairy products, you ingest lactose, a double sugar that must be broken down into two smaller sugars—glucose and galactose—during digestion. It appears that galactose is toxic to the ovaries. The more milk products you consume, the more this potentially toxic substance passes into your bloodstream. Compounding the problem, some women have low levels of a certain enzyme needed to break apart this sugar. For them, galactose builds up dangerously. Its toxic effect on the ovary is reflected in infertility and higher cancer rates. Dr. Cramer and others have confirmed a correlation between the amount of lactose consumed and ovarian cancer rates. For instance, in the Nurses' Health Study, which included 80,326 women, those who consumed the highest amount of lactose (one or more servings of dairy per day) had a 44 percent greater risk for all types of invasive ovarian cancer, compared with those who ate the least (three or fewer servings monthly).

High-lactose foods include skim milk, ice cream, yogurt, and cottage cheese. Yogurt is a significant contributor of galactose to the diet because the bacteria used in its production break apart the lactose before you ever dig in your spoon. In each cup of yogurt you are essentially getting a serving of preformed galactose. So if you have been reaching for yogurt to keep calcium intake up, refer to the list of healthier high-calcium plant foods on page 35, or simply have a calcium-fortified glass of OJ each morning.

Studies have shown that dairy consumed during pregnancy may have long-term health effects for a female baby as well. When a woman has lower levels of the enzyme needed to eliminate galactose, aided and abetted by high levels of lactose in her diet, toxic levels of galactose can harm the development of the baby's growing reproductive organs, which may contribute to endometriosis later in life. More research is needed, but it is well worth being alert to the health effects of dairy products.

Endometriosis

Endometriosis is a disease in which endometrial tissue, which normally lines the uterus, spreads and grows in other parts of the body. During the menstrual cycle, this misplaced tissue swells and bleeds, causing inflammation and pain. Over time this leads to scarring, which can lead to infertility. More than five million women in North America have been diagnosed with endometriosis, about 10 percent of women in their reproductive years.

In a normal menstrual cycle, cells from the uterine lining are shed and passed out of the body at the end of the month. Endometriosis begins when some of these cells slip upward through the fallopian tubes that lead to the abdominal cavity. From there, they can end up attached to the intestinal tract, bladder, or elsewhere. A healthy immune system will normally find and eliminate out-of-place cells such as these. However, in endometriosis, they somehow survive and flourish, causing pain that can be severe, and a gradual loss of fertility.

Avoiding certain foods may add a measure of protection against endometriosis. Although the reasons are not fully understood, caffeine consumption has been linked to the disease. Researchers at the Harvard School of Public Health found that women who have two or more cups of caffeinated coffee (or four cans of cola) per day were twice as likely to develop endometriosis.

Foods that contain polychlorinated biphenyls (PCBs) also tend to encourage endometriosis. As we have seen, these chemicals are most concentrated in animal fat, particularly in fish. In your body, they impair your immune defenses against abnormal cells, including those that have wandered out of the uterus into places where they don't belong.

Animals such as chickens, cows, and pigs are often fed grains that are treated with pesticides or contaminated with organochlorines.

When we eat their meat or drink their milk, we invite these toxins into our bodies, where they can weaken our immune system. Eating organic produce, grown without chemical pesticides, is the best way to get your nutrients in as pure a state as possible. Washing and peeling vegetables and fruits also removes some harmful residues—something that simply can't be done with animal products. What they ingest, to some extent, you ingest, often in a concentrated form.

A prime target for these pollutants is a woman's breast, where they dissolve into the fatty tissue and remain for a very long time. The ultimate victim is a nursing baby, who can receive up to half of all the dioxin a mother has accumulated in her body tissues. By avoiding fish, other meats, and cow's milk, you can greatly reduce organochlorines in the foods you eat. It's no surprise that researchers have found vegetarian women to have much lower levels of harmful pollutants in their breast milk.

Exercise is important as well. Women who work out for just two hours each week have only half the risk of endometriosis as other women. The protection apparently comes from a healthy reduction in hormone activity as well as a boost in immune system functioning.

You will only know for sure whether you have endometriosis after having a medical procedure called a laparoscopy. It allows your doctor to look inside the abdominal cavity through a small incision made below the navel. Current treatments for endometriosis seek to minimize discomfort with anti-inflammatory painkillers. Danazol (a male hormone derivative) is essentially not used any more because of its masculinizing side effects. Gonadotropin-releasing hormone analogs are most widely prescribed, as they effectively shrink endometriotic cells that have gone astray by reducing a woman's estrogen to menopausal levels. However, they are not without risks, and should only be used for up to six months.

Surgical treatments include removing cell clumps or, in severe cases, severing pain nerves, or performing a hysterectomy, which, of course, results in infertility. Surgery and drug treatments have shown similar effectiveness, but usually are temporary measures, as they do not eliminate all of the troublesome cells.

Some women find relief by changing their diet. In the same way that low-fat foods keep estrogen levels in check to help ease menstrual pain, they can keep painful clusters of cells from growing and worsening. A diet change that reduces estrogen can force these cells to wither and die.

Another method for opposing estrogen and reducing endometriosis pain is with natural progesterone, a cream made with wild yams or soybeans. John R. Lee, M.D., a leading expert on women's health issues, recommends that progesterone be used in this instance from day six of the cycle to day twenty-six each month, using one ounce of the cream per week for three weeks, stopping just before the expected period. He cautions that patience will be in order, as it may take four to six months to see results. However, many of his patients, some with no relief from surgery, have had great success with progesterone treatments. His somewhat technical book *Natural Progesterone* is available from BLL Publishing, P.O. Box 2068, Sebastopol, CA, 95473, and addresses the subject in greater detail.

Because endometriosis seems to be caused by an immune-system failure to eliminate out-of-place cells, an immune-boosting diet may help prevent it. That means eating as little fat as possible and bringing in generous amounts of vegetables and fruits. Animal and vegetable fats actually suppress white blood cells' power to annihilate dangerous cells. Cholesterol does the same sort of mischief. When researchers add cholesterol to white blood cells in a test tube, their immune strength is decreased.

Natural immune-boosting foods are easy to find. Orange vegetables are rich in beta-carotene, grains and beans have plenty of vitamin E, and many fruits and vegetables are abundant in vitamin C and other antioxidants. By eliminating animal products and all of their fat and cholesterol, you're giving yourself the best protection possible. When blood samples are studied to see whether certain white blood cells, called natural killer cells, are operating sufficiently, vegetarians do twice as well as omnivores. For them, powerful foods are on the job, protecting every cell.

Polycystic Ovary Syndrome

When women visit doctors' offices to evaluate why they are having trouble conceiving, one of the most common findings is that neither ovary is releasing an egg. Normally, ovulation occurs about two weeks into each monthly cycle. But for some women, no egg is released at all. Month after month, there is no possibility of pregnancy. Most often the cause is a hormonal condition called polycystic ovary syndrome (PCOS), and along with difficulty conceiving come other signs that your hormonal balance is not quite right. You may find masculinizing effects—facial hair or a thinning of hair on your scalp—that can come from a bit too much testosterone, and your periods may be intermittent or may have stopped altogether. You also may find you are having trouble keeping off excess weight.

If you could look at the ovaries, you would see that they are enlarged, sometimes double their normal size, and are studded with cysts, some of which are three-quarters of an inch in diameter. Each cyst is an egg and supporting cells that failed to mature properly for ovulation.

Although for many years doctors have focused on trying to tame the estrogen or testosterone abnormalities found in PCOS, recent studies have shown that the cause is something quite different. The syndrome results from too much insulin. Insulin is a hormone produced in the pancreas, and it helps your body absorb nutrients from the foods you eat. When you take in protein, for example, insulin escorts the individual amino acid molecules that make up the protein chain into the cells of your body, so that your cells can build proteins of their own. When you eat carbohydrates, insulin helps you store their natural sugars for energy. If you have too much insulin in your blood, however, it can wreak havoc with your ovaries. In a moment we'll see how to fix the problem. But first, a brief explanation of what's gone wrong.

First, increased insulin decreases your ability to ovulate. Normally, during your monthly cycle, hormones travel from the brain to the ovaries, triggering the release of an egg and preparing the uterus to receive the embryo. Insulin disrupts these signals. Specifically, it makes the developing eggs mature too rapidly. Like apples or oranges that have ripened well before they reach grocery shelves, the eggs develop out of synch. They are not released and cannot be fertilized.

It appears that nature designed the ovaries to be sensitive to insulin to keep tabs on how well nourished you are. After all, if you are seriously malnourished, it is not a good time to get pregnant. For some women, unfortunately, this system malfunctions, and insulin foils attempts to become pregnant.

And the story gets worse. Insulin also pushes the ovaries to make extra testosterone. Although we associate testosterone with men, women's bodies make it, too, albeit far less than a man's body makes. It has a variety of functions, not the least of which is its responsibility for maintaining your sex drive. The problems start when your testosterone level gets too high.

The first step in treating PCOS is a change in diet. You'll want to cut the fat to the extent you can, boost fiber-rich foods, and select foods that release their natural sugars gradually. Here are the details.

First, cut the fat. Fatty foods make it hard for insulin to do its job. Think of insulin as a doorman who turns the knob on the door to the cells of your body and escorts protein building blocks and sugars inside. When there is too much fat in your diet, insulin becomes very inefficient. It is as if its hand keeps slipping on a greasy doorknob. When this condition, called insulin resistance, develops, your pancreas makes more and more insulin to try to get its job done. This mounting wave of insulin then causes trouble with your ovaries, poisoning their ability to ovulate and pushing them to make too much testosterone.

To avoid fatty foods, the best diets eliminate animal products entirely, which, of course, eliminates all animal fat, and then also keep vegetable oils very low. Research studies show that low-fat vegan diets are very powerful for getting insulin working properly again.

Second, boost the fiber in your diet. High-fiber foods such as whole grains, vegetables, fruits, and beans slow down your digestion and allow for a slow release of sugars from the foods you eat, allowing insulin to do its work more easily. When you have a choice of whole grain bread instead of white bread, or brown rice instead of white rice, go with the high-fiber varieties.

Third, select foods with a low glycemic index. The glycemic index is a tool nutritionists use to choose foods that release sugars slowly. It is calculated by giving foods to volunteers and measuring how quickly their blood sugars rise over the next few hours. It turns out that foods such as white bread that have been stripped of their fiber generally have a higher glycemic index than foods that retain their natural fiber. Processing affects the glycemic index, too. For example, when white flour is compacted into spaghetti noodles, it releases its sugars much more slowly than when it is made into a light and airy loaf of bread.

THE GLYCEMIC INDEX OF VARIOUS FOODS

Fruits

Apple (1, medium)	52
Apple juice (1 cup)	58
Banana (1, medium)	76
Grapefruit (½, medium)	36
Grapes (1 cup)	62
Mango (1, medium)	80
Orange (1, medium)	62
Orange juice (1 cup)	74
Peach (1, medium)	40
Pear (1, medium)	51
Pineapple (1 cup)	94
Watermelon (1 cup)	103

Grain Products

Angel food cake (1 oz)	95
Bagel (1)	103
Barley, pearled (1 cup)	25
Bread, white (1 slice)	100
Bread, whole-meal (1 slice)	99
Bread, rye (1 slice)	92
Bread, pumpernickel (1 slice)	58
Bulgur (1 cup)	68

Grain Products
continued

Cereal, All-Bran (1 cup)	60
Cereal, Cheerios (1 cup)	106
Cereal, corn flakes (1 cup)	119
Cereal, oatmeal (1 cup, cooked)	87
Corn chips (1 oz)	105
Popcorn, air-popped (1 oz)	79
Spaghetti (1 cup)	59
Spaghetti, al dente (1 cup)	52
Rice, white (1 cup, cooked)	81
Rice, brown (1 cup, cooked)	79
Rice, parboiled (1 cup, cooked)	68

Legumes

Baked beans (veg, 1/2 cup)	69
Black beans (1/2 cup)	43
Black-eye peas (1/2 cup)	59
Chickpeas (1/2 cup)	47
Kidney beans (1/2 cup)	42
Lentils (1/2 cup)	41
Lima beans (1/2 cup)	46
Navy beans (1/2 cup)	54
Peas (1/2 cup)	56
Peanuts (1 oz, dry roasted)	21
Pinto beans (1/2 cup)	64
Soybeans (1/2 cup)	25

Vegetables

Carrots (1 cup, boiled)	101
Potato, baked	121
Potato, new	81

Vegetables
continued

Potato chips (1 oz)	77
Spinach (1 cup, boiled)	0
Sweet potato (1, baked)	77
Yam ($\frac{1}{2}$ cup, baked)	73

Sweets

Jelly beans (1 oz)	114
Life Savers (2 pieces)	100
Chocolate (0.5 oz)	70
Honey (1 tbsp)	104
Sugar (sucrose, 1 teaspoon)	92

The lower the glycemic index, the better. Values above 90 or so should be regarded as high. You'll notice that meat products are not included in the table. The reason is that meats are mainly mixtures of protein and fat and do not contain sugars. Some researchers naturally assumed that this meant they would not spark the release of insulin. However, the concentrated proteins in these products cause a very strong insulin release, and they can be your worst enemies when it comes to keeping insulin in bounds.

Fourth, exercise helps. Exercising muscles can draw sugar from your bloodstream with much less insulin than they need at rest. The result is that your body will make less insulin.

Finally, the combination of a change in diet and exercise habits will do one other thing that helps enormously: It will help keep your weight in bounds. Weight loss eliminates much of the excess insulin in your bloodstream, and does the same for excess testosterone. In the process, it brings a return of ovulation for many women.

It is worth emphasizing that the best diet is a low-fat vegan diet. In research at the Physicians Committee for Responsible Medicine and elsewhere, this kind of diet has proven its power in getting blood sugar down, preventing insulin excesses, helping people lose weight easily and effectively, and getting hormones back into balance.

In case you're wondering if a major diet change is worth it, there is one other thing you should know about PCOS. The insulin abnormalities that cause PCOS also lead to an increased risk of other serious health problems, including heart attacks, diabetes, and high blood pressure. A diet change gives you power against all these problems.

The first line of defense is a major change in diet, along with regular exercise. If you need more help, doctors will prescribe medicines that can improve insulin sensitivity and help you rein in hormone actions.

Fibroids

Fibroids occur in about 20 to 30 percent of women over age thirty-five. These noncancerous growths, developing from the muscle cells that provide a layer of strength in the wall of the uterus, can be microscopic or as large as a grapefruit. They are generally harmless, but they can hinder fertility.

A doctor can diagnose fibroids during a pelvic exam or by ultrasound. Additional tests to rule out other conditions may be performed, including a biopsy, a hysteroscopy (using a fiberoptic tube to view the uterus), or a Pap smear. Symptoms of fibroids may include pain and tenderness in the pelvic area, heavy or prolonged bleeding, bleeding between periods, back or leg aches, frequent urination, painful intercourse, or recurrent urinary tract infections.

Although the cause of fibroids is unknown, they appear to be linked to estrogen levels because they tend to grow during pregnancy and shrink after menopause (except when estrogen hormones are taken). A low-fat vegan diet is a powerful estrogen reducer. Taking animal products—and all of their fat—out of your diet in favor of fiber-rich grains, vegetables, fruits, and legumes will dramatically suppress the hormone surges that are at the root of so many reproductive difficulties.

If fertility is an issue for you, by all means see your doctor. There are causes of infertility that have nothing to do with diet, and treatments that require continued medical monitoring.

5

A Healthy, Drug-Free Menopause

In the not too distant past, menopause was quietly referred to as "the change," and it wasn't one that many women looked forward to. It seemed to signify not just the end of fertility but also of youthful vigor. Luckily, those days are largely gone. Today what is changing is our perception of menopause, enabling us to see it for what it is: another normal—even advantageous—biological phase of a woman's life. However, modern women may fall victim to a new, perhaps more harmful, myth—that menopause is not simply a normal phase of life, but a medical diagnosis, one that carries the risks of heart disease, osteoporosis, and inexorable weight gain. One that demands treatment with hormones. One that carries with it as least as many dangers as benefits.

Natural Changes

The world's ever-diminishing borders have expanded our view of how women in other cultures experience menopause, both physically and emotionally. Dietary and lifestyle habits that are common in other countries have allowed many women to breeze through menopause. You can explore and use these insights as well. Not surprisingly, virtually all menopausal symptoms can be alleviated, or prevented entirely, by simple choices we make each day and throughout the years.

Menopause itself is not so mysterious. It occurs for most women between ages forty-five and fifty-five, and simply signifies the time when a woman's cyclic function of the ovaries and menstrual periods ceases. It begins gradually. In fact, related hormonal changes may begin as early as the midthirties. Instead of ovulating more or less regularly every month, you'll miss a month here or there, in what is called an anovulatory cycle. These occur more and more often as menopause approaches. When ovulation does not take place, your hormone balance is tipped a bit. Throughout your adult life up to this point, each monthly cycle has begun with gradually increasing amounts of estrogen, the female sex hormone, in your bloodstream. It thickens the lining of the uterus in anticipation of pregnancy, among myriad other jobs. About fourteen days into the month, an egg is released. Ovulation triggers the production of progesterone, another of your key reproductive hormones, which balances estrogen's actions.

Anovulatory cycles change everything. Without ovulation, progesterone is not produced, and the unopposed estrogen released results in water retention, mood swings, and weight gain. But because menstrual cycles can continue without progesterone, many women—and their doctors—are totally unaware of what's really going on. Estrogen continues its normal cycling, and with no progesterone to balance the effects, symptoms can be miserable.

When menopause does arrive, the ovaries stop releasing eggs altogether and decrease their production of both estrogen and progesterone. Testosterone production, however, can remain at premenopausal levels for a decade or longer. This, along with the estrogen that continues to be made by the adrenal glands and by fat tissues, helps mute the effects of declining hormone production. With testosterone, the hormone responsible for stimulating sexual desire, dominating the hormonal balance, some women say they enjoy sex more after menopause than before. Accompanied by the end of contraception concerns, many women find it to be an ideal time to enjoy a new kind of intimacy and sexual freedom.

It's not all a bed of roses, of course. A reduction in vaginal blood flow may cause less lubrication than before, and the skin that lines the vagina may become thinner and more sensitive to irritation. Hot flashes, mood swings, and anxiety can arrive as well. It's not age, but hormonal *shifts* that cause these symptoms. How healthy you are when these changes come makes all the difference. And, as you will recall, the body is always producing some estrogen from the adrenal glands and fat tissue, if no longer from the ovaries. And nutritious plant foods also provide weak estrogen effects, reducing the chance that such shifts will be great enough to cause bothersome symptoms. Plant-derived estrogen and progesterone creams, along with some surprisingly effective herbs, as we will later see, can alleviate these minor problems as well.

Menopausal Women—Near and Far

Your life experiences have a dynamic effect on how you experience menopause, as is apparent by looking at other countries. For example, in many cultures unaffected by sweeping modern changes, menopause is often a welcome period of liberation from the burdens of menstruation, pregnancy, and child rearing.

An interesting study of menopause in traditional Mayan and Greek cultures was conducted by a medical anthropologist at the University of California. Mayan women, living in the southeastern part of Yucatán, Mexico, still work as traditional subsistence farmers and have not been influenced by Western customs or eating habits. They spend their whole lives eating nutritious, primarily vegetarian, foods such as corn, corn tortillas, beans, tomatoes, squash, sweet potatoes, radishes, and other vegetables. They consume very little meat and no dairy products. As we saw in chapter 3, this very-low-fat diet will reduce the amount of estrogen in their bodies. So while their meat- and dairy-eating counterparts in North America have much more fat in their diets, sparking the production of estrogen, Mayan women are adapted to lower estrogen levels throughout life. When menopause arrives—on average at age 42, several years earlier than in the United States—it simply means that menstruation ceases and fertility has ended. Like Japanese women, they have no word for "hot flash." These and other bothersome symptoms associated with menopause are rare, if nonexistent. How's that for affordable, easy healthcare? Their naturally very-low-fat diet balances hormone levels throughout life.

And there are other reasons why Mayan women welcome menopause. Without readily available contraception, they bear many children. And year after year, they have had to put up with troublesome myths about menses. Menstrual blood is considered an unclean substance of which the body is trying to rid itself, a notion perpetuated by the lack of modern sanitary products. A menstruating woman is also believed to be a danger to others, is not allowed to touch newborn babies, and is thought to bring bad luck to the community by her mere presence. It's no wonder that these women look forward to menopause and the end of such restrictive taboos.

In a village in eastern Greece, women also are considered impure during menstruation. They are barred from participating in church activities or even touching religious icons at home. They must keep their distance from the kitchen for fear food and drink would spoil. After menopause, these burdensome constraints are lifted. And women can enjoy sex with their partners without risk of pregnancy. While hot flashes occur more frequently among Greek women than they do among the Mayans, they are a mild, passing nuisance and not a reason to seek medical attention. Menopause is not only a welcome relief, it is also remarkably free of most of the difficult symptoms troubling women in industrialized societies. Again, the apparent reason is diet. With a diet rich in fruits, vegetables, and bean dishes, there is little fat and plenty of fiber, so a woman's estrogen levels are not artificially elevated. At menopause, estrogen doesn't have so far to fall. A less dramatic decrease makes it less likely for symptoms of "estrogen withdrawal" to occur.

Small diet changes—more vegetables, cutting out the meat—may seem too simple a solution, but it's the accumulated effect that really makes the difference. To put the concept into perspective, note that Western women consume *four times* as much fat and about *half* the fiber, throughout life, as Asian women eating traditional rice-based diets. When most of your calories come in the form of fats, refined starches, sugar, and processed foods, estrogen levels leap to twice those of women in developing countries.

Modern Medicine's Answer to Menopause

If some of the customs in Mexico and Greece seem odd, imagine how women around the world might look upon Western medicine's answer to menopause. In the United States and other developed nations, hormone replacement therapy (HRT) is standard. Menopause is not viewed as a normal phase of life, like losing baby teeth and growing taller, but as a condition that must be masked with drugs if life is to carry on with any normalcy. Many women enter menopause never having realized that their lifelong eating habits were a major contributor to their symptoms, or that there are gentler, more natural ways to ease them along the way.

If you pass through menopause without the use of hormone medications, your hormone-sensitive organs—breasts, ovaries, and uterus—will benefit. Overstimulation of these organs can mean an increased risk for fibrocystic breast disease (causing benign but often painful cysts), uterine fibroids, and even cancer. It is important to note that many physicians *never* prescribe HRT for their patients because they believe the health risks are significant and that there is little sense in masking menopausal symptoms without addresses their underlying causes. The push for HRT that you see on television, in magazines, and even at your doctor's office comes from pharmaceutical companies. Unfortunately, their well-funded campaigns have an impact on all of us, especially doctors.

Under the "menopause as disease" mind-set common in North America, HRT is often hastily prescribed at the earliest signs of menopausal symptoms, along with little information regarding the importance of proper nutrition and other lifestyle habits. A doctor may prescribe estrogen pills or patches, with no more than a word or two about associated risks for uterine and breast cancer. If you've been in this situation, you may also have heard of an increased risk for stroke, blood clots, water retention, breast enlargement, spotting on the skin, irregular vaginal bleeding, gallstones, headaches, and other side effects. And soon you may have felt you were just replacing one set of symptoms with another.

It isn't that menopausal symptoms are not real. For some women, especially those who regularly consume a diet heavy in animal products, symptoms can include hot flashes, depression, irritability, anxiety, shortness of breath, dizziness, fatigue, digestive complaints, sensitive skin, memory lapses, vaginal dryness, muscle and joint pain, and breast tenderness. Of course, each woman's experience is unique, and the number and intensity of symptoms can vary greatly. But drug companies that sell HRT will never tell you about the women who have few menopausal symptoms, or take time to investigate why this is so. Luckily, some physicians have.

Even authoritative educational resources such as *Novak's Textbook of Gynecology* agree that menopause does not signify an "estrogen deficiency" that necessitates HRT. In fact, many medical authorities regard the change as not only harmless but also *protective,* noting how estrogen falls just low enough to prevent reproduction, yet remains high enough to support tissue health. The result is a natural protection against associated growth stimuli that would otherwise occur from continuing estrogen excesses, and that could lead to cancerous growths.

What's *Not* in the HRT Brochure

One of HRT's greatest selling points is its supposed heart-protecting benefits. This has been widely misunderstood as well. Two large studies have confirmed that estrogen replacement therapy does not protect against heart attacks. For the past two decades, doctors have believed that estrogen helps the heart by lowering cholesterol levels and have passed this information on to their female patients. The first major study focusing on this issue followed 2,763 women for four years and found that, if anything, hormones may aggravate heart problems and also contribute to blood clots and gallbladder disease. In a second study, researchers looked at postmenopausal women with heart disease to find out whether HRT slows the buildup of fatty deposits in the heart arteries. No benefits were found.

A popular prescription estrogen called Premarin, made by Wyeth-Ayerst Laboratories, has been aggressively marketed as a "natural" remedy for alleviating menopausal symptoms. It is actually an estrogen collected from pregnant mares' urine. Thus the name "*Pre*gnant *mar*es' ur*ine*." The drug continues to be highly controversial, in part because of its source. In Canada, Minnesota, and North Dakota, thousands of horses are impregnated and confined so their urine can be collected to make the drug. After giving birth, they are reimpregnated, their foals often ending up as meat or joining the herd to furnish future supplies. While Premarin contains estradiol and estrone, your doctor probably won't tell you (and probably doesn't know) that it also contains a large dose of equilin, a horse estrogen that has no natural role in a woman's body.

The U.S. National Toxicology Program lists estrogens used in postmenopausal treatments and birth control pills—including the type found in Premarin—on the nation's list of cancer-causing substances. Scientists have noted their contribution to endometrial cancer and, to a lesser extent, breast cancer.

Osteoporosis protection is HRT's other big draw. However, the dietary and lifestyle measures that significantly reduce bone loss— eating wholesome plant foods, getting moderate exercise and sunlight, and quitting smoking—are so safe and effective that there is no justification for taking cancer-promoting drugs in its place. The biggest hurdle that women face in halting bone degeneration is not their loss of estrogen at menopause. It is simply lack of information. In chapter 10 we will learn how to keep bones strong at any age, in part by avoiding the foods that cause calcium loss and by staying active. For now it is worth noting that osteoporosis should not be viewed as another "estrogen deficiency" disease that is inevitable at menopause. If a bone scan in our fifties or sixties shows bone loss, it almost certainly began long before menopause caused estrogen levels to drop. Although bone loss does accelerate for a few years at menopause, HRT can only slow it, not stop it. And HRT has no ability to rebuild stronger bones. But with the right diet and exercise, and the use of plant-derived progesterone creams if needed, your bones can remain strong—even grow stronger—throughout your life. Just look at chapter 10.

Soy and the Vegan Advantage

Researchers have long observed that Japanese women and men, whose diets have traditionally contained more soy foods, rice, and vegetables than are typical in the West, have far lower rates of breast and prostate cancer. Today, soy foods have gained tremendous popularity in the West in the form of veggieburgers, soy hot dogs, tofu, tempeh, and endless other products. Once found only in health food stores but now available in nearly every supermarket, soy products are in demand. And they have a very useful feature. They contain biologically active phytoestrogens, which are similar to your own natural estrogens but are much weaker. When you eat soy, these phytoestrogens gently occupy estrogen receptors in your body, thus preventing your body's own estrogen from doing so. The result is a reduction in the estrogen stimulation of your cells, and presumably a reduction in cancer risk.

In Asia and other parts of the world where women have long prepared delicious soy, rice, and vegetable dishes in place of fatty animal products, they have enjoyed longer menstrual cycles, meaning fewer menstrual periods. This, and a slightly earlier menopause, mean less lifetime exposure to cancer-boosting estrogen hormones.

The same results have been re-created in clinical studies. In one, women were asked to include soy in their diets for two months, and their menstrual cycles lengthened by an average of 2½ days. In another study, soy protein given over one month blocked estrogen surges, similar to the effects of the cancer-fighting drug tamoxifen. So prior to menopause, soy blocks estrogen excesses. After menopause, when your natural estrogen levels are low, soy's phytoestrogens have a very different effect, actually adding a touch of estrogen to your system. Soy has the amazing effect of regulating estrogen levels; it boosts its effect when your body is low, and suppresses its effect when activity is high. So toss sweet soybeans (edamame) into your next meal, or experiment with soy-centered vegan recipes. Incorporate fresh tofu in a variety of vegetable, bean, and grain dishes a few times each week, or simply ask your favorite Asian eatery to use fresh, steamed tofu in place of beef or chicken in your next order. You won't miss a thing (except the fat). Soy is so versatile; you are bound to find a preparation for it that you'll love. As part of a low-fat vegan diet, it provides a nice supply of vitamins and minerals, so your body can handle transitions such as menopause with greater ease.

Power from Plant Foods

Whether you choose soy products or a natural variety of vegetables, whole grains, beans, and fruits, the plant kingdom will share its medicinal value with you. It's hard to believe that having a breakfast of whole grain cereal instead of eggs, or a dinner of vegetable stew instead of beef stew, can change our lives so profoundly, but individuals and whole populations reaffirm it day after day. When meat is the centerpiece of your meals, you're keeping a steady supply of estrogen-escalating fats pumping through your body. At menopause it's no wonder that the sudden drop from an artificially high level leaves so many women in a state of withdrawal that makes them feel miserable. Women who maintain safe, lower hormone levels throughout life tend to glide into their menopausal years more easily.

No matter when you decide to let foods work to your advantage, you will benefit tremendously. Try new recipes, shop for quick (even frozen) vegan meals at the supermarket, or treat yourself to the culinary delights that vegetarian restaurants now offer. However you choose to begin, just begin. Your arteries will be unburdened from excess cholesterol. Your bones will be protected from the weakening effects of animal protein. And your cells will flourish with nutrients that only plant foods can provide. The earlier in life you begin eating vegetarian foods, the more likely you'll be to enjoy a symptom-free menopause.

Safer Solutions for Persistent Menopausal Symptoms

If you experience menopausal symptoms after changing your diet, there are safer cures than prescription estrogens. First, treat yourself to a brisk walk each day. Walking, or any other kind of exercise, seems to alleviate hot flashes, and puts those mood-elevating endorphins to work. Vitamin E is helpful for some. It should be taken in doses of 400 to 800 IU per day, and not more than 100 IU per day for people with high blood pressure.

Andrew Weil, M.D., a well-known natural health expert, recommends the herbs dong quai, chaparral, and damiana, in capsules or as a tincture. Jesse Hanley, M.D., a family practitioner in Malibu, California, has found that certain Chinese herbs, called Changes for Women by Zand Herbal and Menofem by Prevail, provide relief for some patients. These supplements are available at most health food stores, although you'll want to speak with a herbalist before using any of these compounds.

Although herbs are often marketed as "completely safe" and "all natural," be aware that there are no government regulations imposed on their production or efficacy. While most cause few side effects, use caution when trying an herbal treatment, read labels carefully, speak with knowledgeable healthcare professionals, and listen to your body's signals to determine if it is right for you. Here are several kinds recommended by natural health practitioners.

Dong quai (Angelica sinensis). Used in Chinese medicine for more than two thousand years, this plant from the carrot family is sometimes called the "female ginseng" because of its broad use in balancing women's hormones. Some practitioners prescribe it for irregular menstruation, PMS, recovery after childbirth, and menopausal symptoms.

Caution: It may interact with sunlight to cause rashes. Medical literature indicates it may have a slight estrogenic activity, which dictates that it probably should be avoided in conditions in which higher estrogen levels are undesirable, such as bleeding uterine fibroids or breast cancer.

Black cohosh (Cimicifuga racemosa). The best-studied herb for relieving menopausal symptoms, it appears to work by calming elevated pituitary hormones, specifically luteinizing hormone, which is thought to contribute to hot flashes, insomnia, and depression. Studies have shown a 20 percent reduction in luteinizing hormone in women taking this herb. Other studies have compared symptoms of women taking black cohosh to those taking conjugated estrogens and Valium. The women taking black cohosh reported greater relief of menopausal symptoms and greater reduction in depression and anxiety than people taking the prescription drugs. Further research has found the herb effective in reducing perspiration, headache, dizziness, heart palpitations, ringing in the ears, and sleep disturbances.

Caution: Large doses may cause nausea and vomiting. Because of its possible blood pressure–lowering effects, it should not be used in combination with prescription blood pressure medication.

St. John's wort (Hypericum perforatum). St. John's wort is a natural antidepressant. It works by altering neurotransmitters in the brain. At least ten compounds in the herb may be effective, but hypericum appears to be its most active ingredient. Studies of people with mild to moderate depression have shown the herb to be more effective than a placebo after two to four weeks of treatment, and about as effective as standard antidepressant medications. It should be taken in recommended doses consistently for two to four weeks to assess its effectiveness.

Caution: Do not take St. John's wort with other antidepressant medications. Some people report gastrointestinal upset, dry mouth, confusion, and constipation.

Ginkgo biloba. Traditionally, the Chinese used this herb to treat asthma and bronchitis. It is now licensed in Germany to treat cerebral dysfunction such as memory loss, headaches, and dizziness and is increasingly popular in North America. Ginkgo is believed to improve circulation to the brain, hands, legs, and feet. It has been shown to improve memory in older people, slowing the progression of mental decline. Treatment for four to twelve weeks is usually needed to see results.

Caution: In rare cases, ginkgo may cause stomach upset, allergic reactions, and headache.

Kava (Piper methysticum). Traditionally used as a beverage to induce relaxation, a study of menopausal women found the herb effective in enhancing feelings of well-being and in alleviating depression. In fact, kava has been found to have superior long-term benefits over commonly prescribed antidepressants, with rare adverse side effects.

Caution: Kava may impair motor reflexes. It also may intensify the effects of alcohol. Chronic and heavy use can cause undesirable effects and should be avoided.

Unicorn root (Aletris farinosa). Herbalists use this remedy to alleviate menopausal symptoms, prevent miscarriage, and stimulate menstrual flow.

Hormonal Supplements

If you are considering hormonal supplements, be aware that some preparations may be safer than others. Plant-derived transdermal creams containing the estrogen estriol and smaller amounts of other estrogens are available without a prescription. Current medical evidence indicates that their use probably does not increase cancer risk. Even so, whenever any estrogen creams, including estriol, are used, they should be accompanied by natural progesterone to safeguard against the risk of uterine cancer. Use should be monitored by a physician and tailored to a woman's individual needs.

Transdermal creams containing estriol and other estrogens work by passing through the skin and into the bloodstream, helping to reduce menopausal symptoms. You will need a prescription for pure estriol creams, not because they are risky, but because the process of concentrating them qualifies them as drugs rather than natural preparations.

Natural Progesterone

We've seen how adequate levels of progesterone are essential in a woman's body for many reproductive functions and overall wellbeing. The same is true during menopause. Too little progesterone can contribute to many common symptoms. Ideally, we would all be eating so many healthful plant foods that their natural progestogenic effects would already be at work, facilitating a symptom-free menopause. In many regions of the world this is exactly what happens. Thousands of plants contain sterols that help support healthy ovaries, keeping progesterone levels up, sex drive normal, bones strong, and, in the process, keep menopausal discomforts away.

A long-established progesterone brand called Pro-Gest comes in a transdermal cream. Used for three weeks each month, it gently increases the amount of progesterone in your bloodstream. (See pages 50–51 for more details.) While some manufacturers sell "wild yam cream," their progesterone content usually is too low to be of value.

Putting It All Together

Focus on a good, healthy diet made up exclusively of grains, vegetables, fruits, and legumes—your three-times-per-day opportunity to lower your risk for weight gain, menopausal symptoms, and serious diseases later in life. Also remember that if you are troubled by hot flashes or poor concentration, these symptoms will subside on their own over time. Or you can take advantage of the power of natural herbs. Find activities you really enjoy—ones that get your heart pumping and reduce stress as they allow your mind to take a minivacation. It's never too early; it's never too late.

PART III

Lifelong Health

6

The Keys to
Easy Weight Loss

These days, a woman's size is much more than a number on a scale. For many of us it is deeply entrenched in issues that have as much to do with what's in our heads as on our hips. Body size has become a sort of gauge for personal, sexual, and even intellectual worth. Women—and men, for that matter—who are constantly concerned about weight do not have an easy time of it.

On the one hand, junior high school girls are starving themselves to achieve waiflike thinness. On the other are whole magazines and organizations dedicated to promoting "fat acceptance." And in between are millions of people in a perpetual struggle with every plate of food they consume, wondering why food so easily turns to unwanted body fat. It's a confusing era. We live in a high-tech food chain that, instead of simply providing good, reliable nourishment, bombards us with increasingly unnatural foods in ever-expanding portions. Once we recognize the influences that affect us each day, it is much easier to overcome them.

We're right to be concerned about our collective weight. According to the Centers for Disease Control and Prevention, well over half—now about 60 percent—of American adults are now overweight. This unprecedented epidemic contributes to many of the four thousand heart attacks that occur *every day,* the cancers that eventually hit more than one in three of us, and most cases of high blood pressure and diabetes, diseases that have reached new heights of their own.

Attaining and keeping a healthy body size is not just about appearances, it's also about creating harmony between your mind and your physique. It's about having the freedom to jump from one activity to the next without excess weight holding you back, mentally or physically. It's about protecting yourself from hypertension, heart disease, diabetes, stroke, and cancer. And it's about feeling good, both about the foods you eat and the body they are nourishing. In this chapter we'll get back to nature and see where we got off track.

Why Diets Fail

It's understandable how a high school reunion or a poolside vacation can send you into a panic over unwanted pounds. And it's tempting to dabble with crash diets to shed them quickly. Diets can be effective—albeit unhealthy—for a few weeks or even months. But they are not the way to maintain your ideal weight throughout life. In large research studies, the vast majority of people who lose weight gain it all back—and then some—within a year or two. As you well know, following a "grapefruit diet" or a "cabbage soup diet" for any length of time is totally unrealistic. But the real reason why fad diets fail isn't merely because your taste buds long for a more varied array of foods. They biologically work *against* your natural weight-regulating mechanisms, sabotaging your efforts to trim down.

Researchers at Boston's Children's Hospital found clear-cut evidence that the foods you eat at one meal can affect your snacking later on. They gave teenage boys various breakfasts and then tracked how much they ate later that day. It turned out that those who had had instant oatmeal for breakfast took in 53 percent more snacks later in the day than boys served exactly the same amount of regular oatmeal. The reason: Instant oatmeal has been heavily processed, and it digests very rapidly. It releases its natural sugars a bit too quickly, causing your blood sugar to peak and then plummet, triggering hunger. On the other hand, regular or "old-fashioned" oatmeal is less processed, has its original oat fiber still intact, and releases its natural sugars slowly. There is no big rise and fall of sugar in your blood, and no tendency for hunger to return right after breakfast.

Many dieters seem to have a similar story to tell. They cut way down on food portions and count every calorie, but despite how much weight they lose, it is all gained back again, often more than before. When put on a diet, human bodies are pretty much all the same. They don't care what the "new and improved" diet of the month is, or how important it is for you to look better in shorts. When your body is suddenly deprived of adequate nutrients, it responds as though it is starving. It has two preprogrammed reactions: a slowed metabolism and an increased tendency to binge.

Slowed Metabolism

The first thing to go is your healthy metabolism—your calorie-burning speed. Within just two days of starting a diet, your body will begin to burn calories more slowly—that is, to defend itself against impending starvation and hold on to its fat. In a research study at the University of Pennsylvania, a group of volunteers went on a punishing 420-calorie liquid diet. A month later, the researchers checked their calorie-burning speed, finding it had dropped by an average of 20 percent. That means they were burning about 500 calories fewer each day. Even vigorous exercise cannot counteract this metabolism slowdown that comes from dieting. The worst part is that when you finally come off your diet, your metabolism does not return to normal for several weeks. It stays slow, making it very easy to regain the weight you've just lost. Frustrating as this may be, it is one of nature's life-saving mechanisms to help us outlast periods of food shortages that were common in former ages. Hard as you try to outsmart the system, it's just not possible for very long. The surest way to hang on to the fat you have over the long run is to cut way back on calories and turn down your metabolism.

Genetics does play a part in metabolism, and you may well inherit a tendency toward a rapid or more sluggish rate. However, each bite of food you eat plays a much more significant role in whether your food calories burn up efficiently or hang around waiting to cling to your hips and thighs. Have no fear; you have already learned the secrets to choosing very-low-fat foods (think *plant* foods), and these are just the ones that tend not to turn to unwanted pounds.

Bingeing

The second classic dieting pitfall is the binge. When a diet sends your body into survival mode, it tries desperately to hang on to the fat you have and, naturally, will try to devour every morsel of food that you lay your eyes upon. When your distant ancestors came upon a bounty of food there was no guarantee when the next would arrive, so they took advantage of the opportunity to stock up on calories. Flash forward to today. Although you may have deprived your body of calories for only days or weeks, it will tend to binge when you come upon edible gold mines. When presented with a fat- and calorie-dense plate of cookies, you are virtually powerless to stop with one. This is known as "restrained-eater phenomenon." The easiest way to avoid this automatic binge mechanism is not to restrain yourself in the first place.

Here is how to turn the tables. First, avoid turning on your body's antistarvation devices by eating enough food throughout the day. Make sure that your diet contains at least 10 calories per pound of your ideal body weight. For example, if your goal weight is 125 pounds, your daily menu should contain, at a bare minimum, 1,250 calories. You'll almost certainly need more calories to fuel your day-to-day activities, but if you have fewer calories than this, your metabolism is bound to fall, and you'll be likely to binge. Second, make sure that those calories come from sources that leave you feeling satisfied and provide plenty of vitamins and fiber. Foods that are rich in complex carbohydrates (and naturally low in fat) do just that. Try oatmeal with fruit for breakfast. Eat as many vegetables as you like—carrots, sweet potatoes, spinach, broccoli—prepared without fatty oils or butter, as you will learn to do with recipes included in this book. Treat yourself to new international restaurants where you can try different varieties of pasta, rice, and bean dishes flavored with delicious spices rather than animal fats (one of Western civilization's biggest culinary downfalls). They are all right when you know exactly what you are looking for. For a change of pace, get to know your local Indian, Thai, Ethiopian, or Mediterranean eateries. Restaurants that stick to traditional recipes often have more vegetarian selections, or will gladly substitute tofu or other nonanimal products for meat.

Think of it this way: You will end up eating eventually. Your body will make sure of that. And, in today's society you can't escape coming into contact with giant bags of doughnuts, buckets of chicken wings, and colossal chocolate muffins. *How you are feeling when it happens makes all the difference.* If you just treated yourself to some vegetable lasagna, hearty pasta salad, or lentil soup, you will be able to see these other foods for what they are: a greasy load of fat or sugar (sometimes both). You'll be better able to keep them at arm's length, because you are well nourished.

Where Body Fat Really Comes From

To lose weight and keep it off, you'll want to focus less on *how much* you eat and more on *what* you eat. For most of us, weight on our hips or thighs does not come simply from excess calories. The cause is much more specific, as researchers at a Veterans Administration home in Los Angeles graphically proved. They inserted a tiny needle into the derrieres of a group of volunteers and carefully removed samples of body fat to send to a laboratory. Chemical analysis showed that their body fat did not come from bread, pasta, or potatoes, for the most part. The fat on their bodies mirrored the fats they had been eating. So men who had had plenty of chicken or beef in their diets ended up with remnants of animal fat, almost unchanged, in their own body fat. Those who were keen on olive oil or fried foods had the remains of vegetable fats stored in their behinds. In other words, your body uses the fat you eat to build your own fat layer.

Carbohydrates, whether they are from vegetables, beans, grains, or fruits, actually boost your calorie-burning speed for two to three hours after a meal. They do this by triggering the release of calorie-burning hormones that turn some of the food you've eaten into body heat instead of body fat. Fat in foods does not have the same effect.

So if fat in foods is the cause of our weight problems, where is it all coming from? Animal products, first of all. Meats are simply mixtures of protein and fat, and even the leanest beef, chicken, or fish has more fat than your body needs. Most dairy products (other than the skim versions) are high in fat as well. And oils that have insinuated themselves into French fries, doughnuts, and sauces add to the problem. The most important key to weight loss is to steer clear of these problem foods.

Foods That Make You Hungry

We've all had mornings when we feel hungry barely an hour after breakfast. Or evenings when we're looking through cabinets and refrigerator shelves to cure cravings that linger after dinner. Moments like these can feel devastating to dieters. "How can I be hungry when I just ate?" they ask. It feels as though all of your thoughts revolve around food. There's an easy answer. Hunger doesn't only arise when your stomach is empty; it also occurs when your body isn't properly nourished.

When you eat complex carbohydrates, found in the starchy parts of vegetables, beans, and grains, it takes time for your digestive enzymes to break apart their densely packed molecules. You get a slow, steady release of sugar, and your appetite stays in control. Your energy is more evenly maintained, and your brain and other organs are steadily nourished. However, when you eat refined foods such as white bread, its starches break apart quickly, and sugar rushes through your bloodstream. This rapid rise and fall signals your brain to eat again.

Foods that leave you feeling satisfied the longest include beans, peas, lentils, whole-grain breads such as pumpernickel, certain grain products such as pasta, barley, and bulgur, and vegetables and fruits. Each of these foods has a low glycemic index or GI. They release their nutrients slowly and are your best choices for staying satisfied for hours after a meal. As you can see in the table on pages 61–63, you might try long-grain rice rather than short-grain, and new potatoes instead of russets to fill you up. And don't limit yourself to tiny portions. Prepared correctly, plant foods are very low in fat. They provide a gradual, even burn that will leave you feeling full and satisfied.

"Fake Fats" Fool Your Good Intuition

Your body doesn't long for potato chips; your taste buds do. New innovations in "fake fats" such as olestra, introduced by Procter &

Gamble in 1996, or in reduced-fat ice creams seemed like the answer to dieters' prayers. All taste and hardly any calories. But they had no effect whatsoever on the epidemic of obesity. What these products really do, besides displacing healthy foods and adding unwanted chemicals, is keep your desire for fat turned up high. The more fat—or foods that *taste* like it—you eat all week, the more you'll want tomorrow. A better approach and a worthwhile experiment is to readjust your taste preferences by eliminating the ones that have you captivated. You'll soon see that your preferences are actually determined by what you've eaten in the past three weeks. Just as a person's desire for coffee diminishes after the caffeine addiction is broken, so the desire for fatty, sweet, or, salty foods will lessen—if you give yourself the opportunity. By eating new foods and trying new dishes, you'll awaken your tastes to entirely new flavors. And by consistently reducing the amount of salt and fatty toppings you put on your favorite healthy foods, you'll reeducate your taste buds so that you come to prefer lighter, healthier meals. So skip the "low fat" cheese or "fake fat" potato chips. These foods keep your preferences for fatty foods going strong instead of redirecting them toward more nutritious selections.

Making a clean break of it works best. You can start by mimicking what scientists in Philadelphia discovered: By simply eliminating fatty toppings such as mayonnaise, butter, margarine, and salad dressing, study participants reduced their preference for these condiments. You can, too.

Instead of teasing yourself with unbearably small portions of turkey or chicken, or eating fat-free cheese when you still long for the fat-filled variety, it pays to make a more thorough diet change. In a study by the Physicians Committee for Responsible Medicine and Georgetown University Medical Center, designed to compare various nutritional approaches to controlling diabetes, participants were asked to engage in a total diet makeover. They eliminated all animal products from their diets and used no more than minimal amounts of oil, but ate unlimited amounts of whole grains, fruits, bean and lentil dishes, and vegetables. Most reduced their need for diabetes medications or eliminated them altogether. The average participant lost sixteen pounds over twelve weeks. But a very crucial change came in their feelings about food and eating. Food was no longer the enemy. There was no need to agonize over every bite and calorie, because *the food itself had changed.* The pleasure of eating returned as weight continued to melt away—every dieter's dream come true.

Understanding Genetic Influences

Are you genetically programmed to desire chocolate? Are genes the cause of your Brussels sprouts aversion? Is there something in your chromosomes conspiring against your efforts to slim down? Well, yes and no. You do have built-in calorie-burning mechanisms so that if you have large quantities of fat in your diet, your body has certain methods for handling it. Generally, if you are consuming more fat than necessary, the excess easily turns to body fat. The rare individual may be fortunate enough to stay very thin no matter what he or she eats. In this case, "thin genes" probably dominate the family tree. For example, one study found that about one in every fourteen people has the gene for an unusually rapid metabolism, and it is passed from parent to child. In other families, a gene that causes a slower metabolism can make family members more susceptible to weight gain.

For most of us, however, our genes just make suggestions. More important by far are our eating and exercise habits. Think about professional bodybuilders, for instance. People who commit to a daily weight-lifting routine completely change their body shape. Anyone who might choose to follow their habits would simply be *unable* to maintain their old appearance. This happens for everyone who puts the time in—not to the same exact degree, but it happens. There are no unshakable genetic barriers that will keep you from dramatically changing your body's shape. Weight loss is similar. When you replace tomorrow's chicken breast with vegetable stir-fry over rice and continue, at every meal, to substitute animal products for healthy plant foods, you'll see changes, too—no matter what your genes have to say about it.

When we have trouble losing weight, it's tempting to put the blame on genetics. We figure that if these blue eyes and curly hair came from Dad, this tendency toward an ever-expanding waistline must be his fault, too! Well, science has made great strides in understanding genetic influences in recent years. And it looks, for the most part, as though the ball is really in our court. While your eye and hair color is definitively granted to you at conception, your weight is primarily a result of how you've been treating your body. What may have seemed like an unfair dose of "fat genes" may largely be a legacy of less than ideal eating habits. This is actually good news. If your size and shape were absolutely determined by your genetic makeup, you would be powerless to affect them. In reality, your body is more like a piece of moldable clay—ready and willing to be reshaped whenever you are ready.

This isn't to say that genes are not in the game at all. Science has shown us what their role is—and isn't—as we will see next.

Taste

Tastes are genetic to some extent. Scientists can tell a lot about your food preferences by giving you a little taste of a substance called PROP (6-n-propylthiouracil). It leaves most people with an unpleasant bitterness on their tongue, yet one in four people cannot detect it. Those who can taste it are generally more sensitive to many flavors. For example, too much sugar tastes unbearably sweet, cabbage may taste awfully bitter, and fatty foods may seem over-whelmingly . . . fatty.

Being a PROP-taster may turn you off to sugary drinks, salty snacks, and even alcohol's slight bitterness. Your sensitive taste buds really do taste the foods you eat, so you're more likely to enjoy a meal without needing large quantities. And this is a definite perk. To your disadvantage, you may shy away from any healthy vegeta-bles that trigger your bitter tastes, missing out on their fiber, vita-mins, and cancer-fighting compounds. This does not mean you'll never like vegetables. Tastes change over time. If broccoli hasn't touched your lips for many years, give it another try. You'll find you can actually override your genetic tendencies. Be sure to cook your vegetables adequately and try them over pasta or rice, with flavor-ful new sauces found in the recipes included in this book. A few drops of fresh lemon juice knock the bitterness out of vegetables as well, without adding fat. Fat-free salad dressings provide an endless selection of flavors, too.

PROP-nontasters have virtually the opposite set of challenges. You may gladly eat all your vegetables, then all of your cake and ice cream and perhaps some wine, too. Your "taste blindness" can make it difficult to sense when you have had enough, and you may make up in quantity for what is missing in taste quality. Unfortunately, PROP-nontasters are more likely to gain weight, as Yale University researchers found in a recent study.

Whether you are a PROP-taster or not is purely genetic. There are other predetermined taste preferences, too, and they tend to be similar among genders. Whereas many women are commonly drawn to chocolate, cake, and cookies, men are more often seduced by burgers, fries, and pizza. Whether you are a woman or a man, supertaster or nontaster, you have unique vulnerabilities to face, and if your genes have been nudging you toward the potato chip aisle for far too long, it's time to break the cycle. Understanding your challenges can help you avoid making poor choices.

A Note about Snack Foods

The sweet tooth all children have lingers on for some people, especially women. "Chocoholics" are easy to spot. They may *want* a soda, or *want* a slice of pizza, but they *need* chocolate. It's okay. Although sugar is one of the most common cravings women report, the occasional chocolate bar is not the cause of serious weight problems, and some forms of chocolate are modest in fat. Sweet iced tea or lemonade won't do much harm either. But if your sugar is constantly teamed up with fat in the form of endless candy bars, cake, and ice cream, it is time to readjust your diet to include more filling, fiber-rich foods. The reason why chocolate is favored by so many has never been nailed down, but it is likely its combination of sugar and fat, along with caffeine, a related chemical called theobromine, and an amphetaminelike compound called phenylethylamine.

Whether your love of sweets is genetic or learned, what is important is how it is affecting you today. An occasional chocolate bar is a perfectly fine indulgence, but if you feel controlled by them, or they are adding daily doses of unwanted fat to your diet, there are better ways to manage cravings. Try dessert recipes using applesauce instead of eggs, soy milk instead of cow's milk. Or you can also put sweets aside until you make a total diet change because getting rid of other unhealthy foods during lunch and dinner— hot dogs, omelets, chicken wings—can reduce sugar cravings. The added fiber, antioxidants, and vitamins you'll get from the New Four Food Groups will likely boost your energy, allow you to shed pounds, and benefit your psyche in more ways than you can imagine.

Another seductress to the salivary glands, especially in winter months, is carbohydrates. With shorter days and less sunlight, seasonal depression can occur, elevating your desire to eat bread, cake, and cookies. Carbohydrate-rich foods boost serotonin in the brain, much like antidepressant drugs. Taking advantage of natural antidepressant agents in foods is perfectly healthy as long as you choose wisely. Crusty, whole-grain rolls with jam instead of butter, pasta with zesty tomatoes and garlic instead of cream sauce, or new potatoes with fat-free, spicy salsa instead of sour cream are good for your mind *and* body.

Leptin

You may recall news stories from the mid-1990s that suggested that a cure for obesity had been found. The newly discovered hormone leptin was the momentary superstar because it caused obese laboratory mice to lose weight rapidly. Rodent biology being much different from human biology, the experiments turned up little of value to millions of people looking for a quick way to lose weight, and to the industry hoping to profit by selling it in a pill. Despite this misleading experiment, we do have an understanding of how leptin works in human beings, how genes influence it, and how we can make it work in sync with our weight-loss goals.

Leptin is produced by body fat. As you gain weight and as your fat layer expands, you produce more and more leptin. The increase in leptin acts as a signal to your brain to turn down your appetite. It's a fairly weak signal, however, and obviously doesn't prevent obesity. Nor does adding artificial doses do much at all to help people "trick" their bodies into not feeling hungry, as researchers had hoped. Nonetheless, you definitely want your body's leptin system working normally, because if you lose it, your appetite will go through the roof. Strict dieting easily cuts leptin production and can make your appetite soar.

The way to keep your leptin hormone functioning properly is to eat enough of the right kinds of food. As we saw earlier, it is important to eat the caloric equivalent of ten times your ideal body weight. A goal of 130 pounds indicates a need for a minimum of 1,300 daily food calories, and almost certainly more. Going on a calorie-restricted diet will cause your leptin to fall quickly, causing an appetite rebound. Refocusing your attention toward *what* you eat, and not *how much,* will allow your leptin to work for you.

LPL

LPL or *lipoprotein lipase* is also partly determined by your genetic makeup. This critical enzyme decides whether the fat you eat will be stored on your body or be burned off for energy. LPL is found in the small blood vessels that course through your body fat. As particles of fat move by in your blood, LPL pulls them out and adds them to your fat layer. The same LPL enzymes work similarly in your muscles, sliding fat in and burning it up for energy to fuel your movements. This is where genes play a role. Many cases of overweight reflect a predisposition to store fat. Do you have any say in the matter? Yes, you do. If you add a steady consumption of high-fat foods, weight gain can creep up quickly. If your body stores fat a bit more easily than the next person, it is critical that your food choices give your cells little to work with—not little food, *little fat.*

German researchers found that one in thirty obese people carries a gene that turns other cells, called fibroblasts, into fat cells. But for the rest of us, it's merely a matter of how much fat we give LPL to work with. Everyone's LPL works the same way in that it is always looking for fat in the diet. LPL doesn't pick up carbohydrates or proteins and turn them into fat. It locates the fat you consume in your steak, chicken breast, fish sandwich, heavy salad dressings, or breakfast sausage and, with little chemical transformation, delivers it right into the cells of your body. Although we do need traces of fat in our diet for important biological functions, the requirement is just *one-tenth* the fat that most of us actually consume.

Insulin

Your genes also make the hormone insulin. Insulin's job is to escort nutrients—sugar and protein in particular—from the bloodstream into the cells of your body, where they can be used. When insulin is working right, it can be your best friend as you aim to trim off the pounds because, when insulin brings sugar into your cells efficiently, it can be burned as energy. This "after-meal burn" is responsible for 10 percent of all the calories you burn in a day, without lifting a finger.

Your after-meal metabolism boost depends on two things: the foods you eat and the health of your insulin. Pasta and other grain products, vegetables, and beans deliver a powerful burn because their healthy complex carbohydrates deliver natural sugars that are easy to convert to energy. Foods high in fat, such as meat or eggs, do not. They have a load of fat that simply gets stored in your body. Healthy insulin gets nutrients into your cells, but when it is impaired by eating too many greasy foods and accumulating too much body fat, it can't perform well at all. In medical terms this means that your cells are becoming resistant to insulin. And here's the problem. If your insulin isn't working well, your body makes more and more of it to overcome the cell's resistance. When insulin is at work, it temporarily shuts down your fat-burning machinery. So if your insulin is constantly working overtime, you can see how this can easily lead to weight gain.

Your goal is to make your insulin efficient so it can get sugar into cells fast without shutting down your fat-burning machinery for very long. To increase your insulin's efficiency, you can do two things: Cut the fat from your diet, and increase your daily activity. When you get the grease out of the foods you eat, insulin can start working properly again.

Movement—the Essential Sculptor

To further increase your insulin sensitivity, keep moving. If you are new to exercise, simply start walking. Start casually, perhaps three times per week. As you get in better condition you can walk more briskly for longer periods of time. Walking is great for people at nearly any fitness level. Dancing, swimming, cycling, or playing tennis will tone your muscles, increase your energy, and tame your appetite, providing yet another barrier to weight gain. The endorphins released by your brain during aerobic exercise also elevate your mood to keep you on the right track toward total fitness.

Here are some common exercise activities, with the number of calories they burn for a 150-pound adult. For a 100-pound person, subtract one-third. For a 200-pound person, add one-third.

HOW MANY CALORIES WILL I BURN?

A brisk half-hour walk	220
A leisurely half-hour bicycle ride	120
A half-hour bicycle ride at moderate speed	200
A half-hour leisurely swim	140
A half-hour fast swim	250
A slow half-hour jog	370
A quick half-hour jog	460
Running in place for half an hour	325
A half hour of singles tennis	200
A half hour of cross-country skiing	350
Jumping rope for half an hour	375

From This Day Forward

Whether you are twenty, thirty, or eighty pounds too heavy for comfort, or you are simply weary of counting each calorie to maintain your figure, switching to the New Four Food Groups is the safest, healthiest way to go. For the most noticeable results, both in weight loss and increased energy, give it 100 percent. You wouldn't ask your doctor for "a mediocre weight-loss plan for partial success." You'd want the best for yourself. The only way to eat for weight loss or maintenance without robbing yourself of vital nutrients is by eating generous portions of low-fat, fiber-rich foods. In research studies at the Physicians Committee for Responsible Medicine, doctors throw out animal products completely and keep vegetable oils very low. And study participants are inevitably surprised at how easily they lose weight. Most likely, with minor adjustments to your routine, you'll see that this kind of change is much, much easier than thinking in old-fashioned terms of portion size and weight. Forget about calories, forget about restrictions. Enjoy food and lose weight.

7

Cancer Prevention

What would you think if you looked out your window and saw a traveling "lung cancer detection" trailer? In no time at all, a health-care worker could screen you for early signs of lung cancer, quite possibly saving your life. Not a terrible idea, you might conclude, but not exactly hitting the mark. After all, we already know that smoking is the single most important risk factor for developing lung cancer. And we know that arming the public with this infor-mation has saved countless lives. Wouldn't our resources be better spent bolstering programs that keep people from smoking, and pre-vent the disease in the first place? Of course they would. And in the case of lung cancer, we are doing just that.

If the same resources had been poured into aggressive breast cancer prevention programs—not just early detection—we might actually be winning the "war on cancer," which was declared back in 1972 but has yet to make a real difference in the lives of most women. Instead, we've taken a turn for the worse. In the first two decades after the "war" was declared, breast cancer rates climbed inexorably and have only recently begun a modest decline. Breast cancer now strikes one in eight women, up from one in fourteen women just thirty years ago. For lack of better life-saving strategies, many women are resolved to do nothing more than having yearly mammograms after age forty, waiting for the one that reveals cancer, hoping to destroy it before it destroys them. Not exactly a decisive "war tactic," nor a blueprint for good health any mother could confidently pass along to her daughters. Programs that focus solely on early detection strategies ignore all we know about prevention.

When it comes to lung cancer, everyone has gotten—if not heeded—the message: Give up cigarettes. With other types of cancer, we've been much slower to shun equally harmful culprits—poor diet, inactivity, environmental factors, and certain medications—that are strongly linked to causing the disease. We cannot pinpoint the exact cause of breast cancer in individual cases, nor can we prevent it 100 percent of the time. But we do know of risk factors so strongly associated with its development that taking steps to eliminate them can almost certainly lower your risk.

One way that the government evaluates progress in its war on cancer is by looking at "five-year survival" rates, that is, the number of patients who are living five years after being diagnosed with cancer. When these rates improve, the news hits the media, and we feel as though we are approaching a cure. The unfortunate truth is, we are just finding it sooner.

A recent study in the *Journal of the American Medical Association* pointed out that five-year survival is more likely today because patients are often diagnosed when the tumor is small. This is not to say that better treatment methods are not prolonging the lives of those with cancer and many other diseases. But treatments still have a long way to go and, most important, chemotherapy and cancer drugs are not *stopping* the disease from occurring. Researchers examined data on twenty types of cancer diagnosed between 1950 and 1995, looking at incidence, five-year survival, and mortality. Although five-year survival rates increased for all twenty cancers, *occurrence decreased for just five.* The study authors argue that policymakers should focus on mortality rates, the truest indicator of whether we are defeating cancer or any other life-threatening illnesses. With a more accurate measure of progress, perhaps more effective cancer prevention initiatives would be developed. As it stands, five-year survival shows little relationship to overall mortality rates, which is what really counts.

Understanding Risk Factors

The key to living a long, healthy life, and protecting yourself and your family, lies in understanding a few risk factors. A risk factor is anything that increases a person's chance of getting a disease. It's clear to most people that a high cholesterol level is a risk factor for heart disease and that prolonged exposure to direct sunlight is a risk factor for skin cancer. Simply having a risk factor for a cancer—or any other disease—doesn't mean that you will necessarily develop it. Likewise, disease can occur even when no known risk factors can be identified. However, our best scientific evidence shows that 70 to 80 percent of all cancers can be attributed to lifestyle factors such as the foods we eat, whether we smoke or drink alcohol, and whether we are physically active. These are risk factors that are within our control. Only a small minority of cancers appear to be associated with environmental pollution, or the hereditary factors or "cancer genes" we have heard so much about in recent years. In fact, even when cancer-susceptible genes are present, diet and lifestyle contributions can play a crucial role in whether they are ever expressed.

Breast Cancer Today

Breast cancer is the second most common cancer found in North American women, excluding nonmelanoma skin cancers. Prominent cancer organizations address risk factors in term of those that are "set" or unchangeable, such as sex and gender, and those that we can alter, such as diet and smoking. But before you become discouraged by what seems like a long list of fixed risk factors, take note that there is often a fine line between set and alterable risk factors. For instance, your age is beyond your control, but your health and fitness level as you enter your fifties, sixties, or seventies is profoundly affected by lifelong dietary and other habits.

"Set" Risk Factors

Gender, age, and race. It's no surprise that being a woman makes breast cancer more likely. Breast cancer does occur in men, but it is nearly a hundred times more common in women.

If you listen to cursory medical reports, simply aging can seem like a scary prospect. You'll often hear that more than three-fourths of women who are diagnosed with breast cancer are over age fifty. This drives the push for yearly mammography for women in this age group. But a look at breast cancer rates in women over fifty in countries such as Thailand, Japan, Taiwan, Mexico, and the Philippines, which are extremely low, reveals that breast cancer is not necessarily a disease of old age, but may often reflect accumulated lifelong habits, not the least of which is diet.

Caucasian women are slightly more likely to develop breast cancer than African American women, while Asian, Hispanic, and Native American women have a slightly lower risk.

Radiation. Radiation can damage DNA, causing cell mutations that can lead to cancer. Women who have had chest radiation therapy as a treatment for another type of cancer have an increased risk for breast cancer.

While X rays are an invaluable diagnostic tool, they tend to be overused. There is no completely safe dose of radiation, and your risk for cell damage accumulates with each exposure. Any amount of radiation, however small, adds to your total risk. If your physician suggests X rays, be sure you have a clear understanding of why they are necessary.

Many women may not realize that mammograms are X rays, too. While they can be life-saving, you'll want to be certain that modern, low-dose (1 rad or 1,000 millirads) equipment will be used. As the age recommendation for yearly mammograms has steadily decreased (it is currently for women forty or older), it's important that women know about associated risks and about prevention before making this decision.

Radiation also comes from natural and manmade sources, such as uranium or nuclear power plants. Working in particular industries such as radiology, nuclear power, mining, or in any field that exposes you to ionizing radiation increases your exposure. Even common items such as luminous wristwatches, smoke detectors, chinaware, eyeglasses, and dental porcelains can contain radioactive materials.

Women going in for a mammogram may not recognize how common it is for the results to be deemed "suspicious" upon initial viewing. Surprisingly, a new study published in the *Journal of the National Cancer Institute* found that women face a nearly 100 percent chance of having a false positive result at some point in their first nine routine mammography screenings. Some "suspicious" masses are later diagnosed simply as cysts or swollen glands. This can lead to unnecessary biopsies and further radiation (from additional mammograms) as well as needless anxiety for many women.

Researchers found that false positive readings increased with the number of past breast biopsies, family history of breast cancer, estrogen use, length of time between mammograms, lack of previous mammography (for comparison), and the radiologist's individual tendency to call mammograms abnormal. Only increasing age was related to a decreasing chance of a false positive test. Hopefully, understanding the high chance of receiving a false positive result will help reduce fear if the physician recommends further tests. However, the study also underscores the trouble, in general, with depending solely on early detection for saving women's lives. As we will see in more detail below, preventive strategies through lifestyle modifications should be the priority in the fight to defeat this disease.

Previous breast cell growth. Fibrocystic changes without proliferative breast disease or "fibrocystic breast disease," the widely used but somewhat misleading term used to describe multiple symptoms such as pain, swelling, lumps, and discharge, is not associated with breast cancer risk at all. However, if an earlier breast biopsy was found to show intraductal hyperplasia (literally meaning "too many cells in the duct"), if these cells begin to look irregular (intraductal hyperplasia with atypia), or if the cells continue growing and clogging up the ducts in the breast (ductal carcinoma in situ), the risk for breast cancer looms. All three are reversible, and close follow-up by a physician is essential.

Personal and family history. Breast cancer risk is higher among women whose close blood relatives have had the disease, and for those who have had it previously themselves. Some cancer researchers report that having a mother, sister, or daughter with breast cancer doubles a woman's chances of getting it herself. Being in this category can make a woman feel powerless to prevent it. However, it is important not to overlook the fact that lifestyle habits such as diet, exercise, smoking, and drinking are often shared among family members, falsely giving the impression of inherited risk. Therefore it is especially important, if you fall in this category, to adopt a cancer-prevention lifestyle, as outlined subsequently.

Menstrual periods. Women who begin menstruating early in life (before age twelve) or reach menopause at a late age (after fifty) have a slightly increased risk for breast cancer, presumably because of greater lifetime exposure to estrogen. We think of these life stages as "fixed"; however, they are strongly influenced by diet. As we saw in chapter 3, the age of puberty is strongly affected by nutritional factors, as is the age of menopause. Learning this as an adult can be frustrating because you can't go back and change your age of puberty. However, the right kind of diet makeover *at any age* can change the course of development for many diseases, including cancer. Starting your own children on the best nutritional path early, providing a wholesome variety of vegetables, fruits, and other vegan foods, will give them a priceless head start.

Genetics. Although much has been learned in recent years about *how* genes influence cancer development, it appears that fewer than 10 percent of breast cancer cases are hereditary. Scientists have come to learn how certain faulty genes, called BRCA1 and BRCA2, are unable to prevent cells from growing abnormally. Today women can have a genetic blood test to determine whether they have inherited the BRCA1 or BRCA2 genes. Still, there is no changing your genetic makeup, so it is still essential to adjust your diet and lifestyle to lower your risk as much as possible. Remember that most DNA mutations that drive breast cancer occur during a woman's life rather than having been inherited. Considering that more than 180,000 women in the United States will be diagnosed with breast cancer this year, we can assume a staggering 160,000 women became ill at least in part because they didn't know about the many ways to help prevent it.

Risk Factors You *Can* Control

Diet. The foods you eat throughout life have an important effect on lifetime cancer risk, both because of their ability to adjust your hormone balance and because of their effect on body weight, which is strongly associated with risk for breast cancer, especially after menopause. Cutting fatty foods—meat, dairy, eggs, fried and oily foods—is priority number one when you endeavor to lower your risk for beast cancer. As fat in your diet falls, so will the amount of estrogen in your bloodstream. In turn, this dip in estrogen will stop the overstimulation of cells in your reproductive organs. Furthermore, getting rid of cholesterol reduces yet another fuel for cancer-cell growth. Avoiding both animal and vegetable fats strengthens immunity to stop the spread of cancer.

But cutting the fat is just half the story. When researchers first observed lower rates of breast cancer in Japanese women, they soon realized that their low-fat diet deserved much of the credit, but that wasn't all. It's now clear that generous amounts of vegetables and soy foods in the traditional Japanese diet provide many more antioxidants and phytochemicals (the natural cancer-fighters found in all plant foods) than we get from filling up on chicken or fish. This highly protective combination—low-fat and vegetable-rich—keeps cancer away. Unfortunately, today's Japanese women, who are changing their diets with the influx of high-fat foods into their country, are experiencing greatly increased rates of breast cancer. The lesson is clear: If genetics is on their side, or yours, it's still no match for the effect of diet.

You can easily protect yourself in the same way. Eliminating animal products from your diet will dramatically cut the fat and remove all the cholesterol, making room for nutrients that restore and repair cells, slow the aging process, and prevent disease. Antioxidants and phytochemicals, which directly inhibit cancer formation, are concentrated in whole grains, vegetables, beans, and fruit. The antioxidant lycopene, found in tomatoes, watermelon, strawberries, and other bright red plant foods, is a potent cancer fighter. So bake your tomatoes and try them over polenta with black olives and fresh garlic instead of putting them on a hamburger, and you'll boost your cancer protection and also avoid dangerous heterocyclic amines, the cancer-causing toxins that form as meats are grilled.

Foods do much more than provide protective nutrients. They can change your basic biochemistry and adjust your hormones in surprising ways. An optimal anticancer diet keeps a woman's estrogens low, just as the powerful drug tamoxifen was designed to do. A safe and inexpensive way to mimic this effect, without the risk of dangerous side effects, is by eliminating the foods that drive estrogens up. Getting away from meat, eggs, and dairy products will eliminate animal fats completely. The American Cancer Society recommends "limiting your intake of high-fat foods, particularly those from animal sources." And when you not only limit, but *eliminate* them altogether, you can easily double and triple up on those nutrients proven to promote health. When you avoid animal products, use cooking oils sparingly, and learn to prepare savory, oil-free recipes such as those at the back of this book, you're living a cancer-prevention lifestyle.

One additional benefit of healthy foods is their ability to help you eliminate chemicals from your body. Toxic substances that assault your cells and stimulate the release of free radicals are everywhere—in the air, water, and food. Inside your liver are enzymes designed to annihilate them before they cause you all sorts of harm. Their effectiveness depends greatly on the foods you eat. The best way to power up on these enzymes is by eating plenty of vegetables, especially cruciferous varieties such as broccoli, cabbage, Brussels sprouts, kale, and cauliflower. They are able to fight off a variety of chemicals, even those relatively new to mankind such as automobile exhaust and factory fumes. This is important because we cannot avoid all exposures to toxins or know exactly which ones we breathe in daily, but we can prepare our cells with substantial armor.

Oral contraceptives. Large studies have found that women who use birth control pills, especially older formulations taken at a young age and for many years, have a slightly higher risk for breast cancer unless use is discontinued for ten or more years.

Hormone replacement therapy (HRT). We already know that breast cancer is a hormone-driven disease, meaning estrogen encourages cancer cells to grow rapidly (and perhaps start in the first place). Therefore it is logical to avoid drugs such as HRT that add more. Research has shown that breast tumors grow more rapidly with estrogen stimulation and shrink when estrogen is reduced. Avoidance of HRT, in combination with a low-fat vegan diet, brings estrogen levels down to the safest level possible.

Alcohol. For the best protection against breast cancer, it's a good idea to stick to nonalcoholic beverages. Alcohol inhibits the liver's ability to detoxify cancer-causing substances in the blood, weakens the immune system's ability to repair damaged DNA, and raises estrogen levels. Studies have shown that just one drink per day can raise breast cancer risk by as much as 50 percent. Alcohol drinking also is associated with cancers of the esophagus, mouth, and throat.

Physical activity. Exercise is beneficial for many reasons, not the least of which is lowering breast, uterine, and cervical cancer risk, possible by lowering excess levels of estrogen. Engaging in sports, classes at the gym, seasonal activities such as snow skiing or swimming, and even daily walking boosts your immune system, not to mention its value in alleviating negative moods.

Weight. Not only does trimming the pounds cut the risk that cancer will occur, but when it does occur, slimmer women tend to live longer than women with more body fat. As we saw in chapter 6, the best way to slim down is to focus on the type of food you eat, not on the amount. Following a low-fat vegan diet is an easy, life-long way to maintain a healthy weight. The best part about it is that it's not really a "diet" at all. Delicious vegan foods are naturally low in fat, so quantity and calorie restrictions are no longer the focus. Pounds often melt away effortlessly.

Breastfeeding. Some studies suggest that breastfeeding may slightly lower breast cancer risk, especially if it is continued for $1\frac{1}{2}$ to 2 years. Other studies found no effect on breast cancer risk.

Uterine and Ovarian Cancers

Cancers of the uterus and ovary are similar to breast cancer in that sex hormones, and the foods that elevate them, play a role in their development, and both are rarer among those who follow a low-fat, plant-based diet. Women who avoid overweight also are at lower risk. Estrogen supplements used in hormone replacement therapy can increase uterine cancer unless progesterone is added to the regime.

Foods play an important role in cancer of the ovary, too. Not only does it help to avoid fatty foods; adding vegetables and fruits provides a measure of protection. Yale University researchers found that two small vegetable servings per day can lower risk by 20 percent. Every 10 grams of saturated fat in a woman's daily diet increases her risk of ovarian cancer by 20 percent. That is the amount in 2 glasses of whole milk or just 2 ounces of cheddar cheese.

Dairy products may play a special role in ovarian cancer. In addition to whatever fat they contain, they also have lactose sugar. As lactose breaks down in the body, it releases galactose, which is believed to be toxic to a woman's ovaries. Harvard researchers have found not only that the diets of women with ovarian cancer tend to be higher in dairy products, but also that the same appears to be true for women with infertility (as we saw in chapter 4).

Oftentimes, scientists are wary to declare causes of cancer until evidence is too strong to be ignored. This was true of lung cancer and smoking, and the same trend has occurred with female reproductive cancers. Even now we can't assert that every smoker who gets lung cancer got it from smoking. But when it comes to disease prevention, its associations to diet, alcohol use, and other factors are extremely valuable pieces of the puzzle. Extensive population studies have shown us that lifestyle factors drive breast cancer. We have a clear enough idea of what they are, and there is no need to wait for researchers to announce it on the evening news. Our daily habits, from eating and drinking to exercise and prescription drug use, play a role in the health of your cells—breast cells, ovarian cells, every cell. Each habit can work for you or against you, giving you more power for health than you may have ever imagined.

8

Protecting Your Heart

Your heart is a fragile thing. Not much bigger than your closed hand, it sends blood and oxygen to every part of your body. At the end of a long, hard workday, when your tired arms and legs get a well-deserved rest, your heart keeps on pumping, never taking a break. A surprising number of people give their bodies a real beating with unhealthy foods, smoking, and stress. And their hearts cannot take it. In Western countries, heart attacks are the leading cause of death, and the same trend is beginning in developing countries as well.

In this chapter we'll look at how to give your heart the tender, loving care it deserves. But before we go any further, there is a disturbing fact you should know: Almost everything you have learned about keeping your heart healthy—whether you heard it from your doctor or read it in a well-meaning article in a health magazine—is wrong. Most of the information out there about diets, the value of hormone replacement, and even how to interpret your cholesterol test is outdated and inaccurate unless you are one of the lucky few to find an information source linked to the latest research. There are now more powerful ways to keep a healthy heart than doctors dreamed of not too many years ago, and you can put them to work today.

A New Approach Emerges

You arrive at your doctor's office asking for advice about keeping your cholesterol down. Or perhaps your doctor is offering it without your having to ask. The "heart healthy" diet most physicians prescribe comes from what is called the National Cholesterol Education Program, a federal program based, unfortunately, on research conducted a couple of decades ago. As first glance, the diet seems reasonable enough. It advises you to shift your menu from red meat to white meat, remove the skin from chicken, choose leaner cuts, and switch from whole milk to skim. In the mid-1990s, however, researchers put this diet to the test. It turns out that it barely lowers cholesterol levels at all. Even with strict adherence, this chicken-and-fish diet reduces the amount of cholesterol in your blood only about 5 percent—not nearly enough to prevent heart problems. Even more troubling is the fact that when researchers looked inside the arteries of people who followed this diet for several months, they found that artery blockages got worse, not better.

Another common approach used by many doctors is to prescribe estrogens, usually in combination with progesterone for women after menopause. Indeed, some early research studies hinted that hormone replacement therapy, or HRT, might reduce the risk of heart problems for some older women. But new research has made many of them tear up their prescriptions. Careful studies have shown that women on HRT have as many heart attacks as other women and actually seem to have them a bit sooner. And when it became clear that HRT also boosts breast cancer risk, many women began looking in earnest for a better way to stay healthy.

And it has arrived. A Harvard-trained physician named Dr. Dean Ornish started a series of research studies with an ambitious goal. He wanted not only to prevent heart disease but also to reverse it. And he aimed to do it not with drugs or surgery but by prescribing simple changes in diet and lifestyle. Could this kind of program be powerful enough to rejuvenate arteries blocked by years of unhealthy diets, smoking, and stress?

To find out, Dr. Ornish invited heart patients in the San Francisco Bay Area to come to a series of evening classes where they would learn how to make powerful lifestyle changes. They wouldn't just cut their cholesterol intake. They would learn how to virtually eliminate cholesterol from the foods they ate. They traded red meat, chicken, and fish for an entirely vegetarian menu. Roast beef was replaced with spaghetti marinara; creamy soups were swapped for minestrone, lentil, black bean, or split pea soup; and hamburgers became veggieburgers. If they smoked, they had to stop. They began a regimen of daily walks, and learned how to cut stress.

One year later, everyone had an angiogram, a special X ray that shows blockages in the arteries that nourish the heart. The results made medical history. A comparison group of patients who followed more typical medical advice showed that, as expected, their artery blockages continue to worsen, eventually leading to heart attacks. But for patients who made the diet and lifestyle changes, artery blockages not only stopped getting worse; they were actually starting to go away—so much so that the research team found a measurable difference in 82 percent of the patients in the first year. It was as if time were going backward. Even stubbornly clogged arteries began to open up, letting more and more blood pass through to the heart muscle. Five years later, Dr. Ornish again tested the patients, and their progress continued.

For many patients, the diet and lifestyle change was a total revelation. They felt better than they had in years. They had energy like teenagers. And, perhaps best of all, they lost a considerable amount of weight. The average participant lost more than twenty pounds in the first year, without counting calories or avoiding seconds at mealtime.

But Will It Work for Women?

One issue was not solved by this early research study: Will it work for women? Most of the original participants were men. And just as heart problems tend to occur at older ages in women, they might be more resistant to the effects of diet and lifestyle changes, too. An important new piece of information came from research done by Dr. Neal Barnard and his colleagues at the Physicians Committee for Responsible Medicine in Washington, D.C., some of whom are on the expert panel producing this series of books. Dr. Barnard tested a diet similar to that used by Dr. Ornish in a group of thirty-five women. The result: Their cholesterol levels plummeted. In fact, the cholesterol-lowering power of the diet was the greatest ever reported in premenopausal women—three times greater than that achieved with the National Cholesterol Education Program diet.

Was the diet difficult or austere? Not at all. It did require learning a new trick or two in the kitchen, but it was very doable. And a follow-up report in the *Journal of Nutrition Education* showed that women liked the new menu at least as well as their normal diet.

It turned out that people who are dissatisfied with their diets are not those who make healthy diet changes but rather those who are prescribed weak and ineffective diets. They would like to lose weight and see their cholesterol levels drop, but their diets just don't do the job. Weak diets—like the old-fashioned ones most doctors still use—are exercises in frustration. Diets that do what they are supposed to are a joy.

What Is Cholesterol, and How Does It Hurt the Heart?

Before we look at a healthy diet in detail, let's make a quick review of what heart disease is and how nutrition affects it.

Your heart needs a good blood supply to carry oxygen to its hardworking muscle cells, just as your arms, legs, brain, and internal organs need wide-open blood vessels to function. And arteries that ring the heart like a crown, called coronary arteries, provide it. They dive into the muscle tissue, branching out to supply every cell in the heart with the nutrients they need.

For many people these arteries are gradually becoming constricted. First, a yellowish fatty streak appears on the artery's inside wall. Eventually small bumps, called plaques, form from cholesterol, fat, and overgrowing cells, narrowing the passage for blood flow. Eventually they can block the artery enough to cause pain, which doctors call angina. If a portion of the heart muscle dies, this is a heart attack, or myocardial infarction.

The foods you eat are critical, and the key issue is cholesterol. A small amount of cholesterol is normally made by your liver, which sends it into your bloodstream to act as a raw material to build hormones. Your body uses cholesterol to make estrogen, progesterone, testosterone, and other compounds. Cholesterol also is delivered to the cells of the body, where it acts as a kind of cement that holds the cell membranes together.

The problems start when there is too much cholesterol in your blood. With too much of this "cement" in your bloodstream, it ends up where it doesn't belong—irritating the walls of the arteries, causing plaque to form.

And here is where foods come in. Chickens, fish, cows, and all other animals have livers, just as you do. Their livers are busily making cholesterol, too, which is packed into their meat, milk, eggs, and any other animal tissue. If you include these products in your diet, some of the animal's cholesterol adds to your own.

Here are the numbers: Every 100 milligrams of cholesterol on your plate as part of your daily routine adds about 5 points to your blood cholesterol level (i.e., 5 milligrams per deciliter, or 0.1 millimole per liter for those using international measurements). If you were to start your day with, say, an egg for breakfast, you've added over 210 milligrams of cholesterol to your diet. A skinless half chicken breast for lunch adds 75 more. A shrimp dinner easily adds another 150 milligrams, adding up to 435 milligrams for the day. Doing this daily adds 20 points to the average person's cholesterol level.

There are about 100 milligrams of cholesterol in 4 ounces of beef, 4 ounces of chicken, 3 cups of whole milk, or in just ½ egg. You might be surprised to learn that chicken has essentially the same amount of cholesterol as beef. Chicken can be slightly lower in fat, but fat and cholesterol are two separate issues.

Skip the Chicken Fat

Certain types of fat stimulate the liver to manufacture more and more cholesterol, and it is easy to tell which ones they are. The problem fats are those that are solid—such as butter, chicken fat, or beef fat—as opposed to liquid vegetable oils. Animal fats are solid because they are loaded with *saturated* fat, and that is what stimulates your liver to make cholesterol. Vegetable oils, on the other hand, are rich in *unsaturated* fats, which do not have this effect.

For people who like technical explanations, the term "saturated fat" refers to the fact that each fat molecule is completely covered —saturated—with hydrogen atoms, which makes the fat waxy and solid. This kind of fat tends to raise your cholesterol level. Vegetable oils are rich in unsaturated fats, meaning there are fewer hydrogen atoms in the mix. They are liquids at room temperature and will not raise your cholesterol. When hydrogen atoms are chemically added to liquid oils, however, the resulting hydrogenated fats are similar to animal fats in their effect on your cholesterol level.

From the standpoint of cholesterol, plant oils are much healthier than animal fats. Nonetheless, there are a few oils you should be wary of. Tropical oils (coconut, palm, and palm kernel oil) are unusual in that they are high in saturated fats. Sometimes they turn up in commercial baked goods or snack foods. Likewise, many snacks and baked goods are made with hydrogenated vegetable oils, which have been chemically altered by the manufacturer and can increase your blood cholesterol level.

Here's the take-home message: The most powerful heart-conditioning diets use vegetarian foods and avoid animal products completely. All animal products—poultry, fish, beef, eggs, and dairy products—contain both cholesterol and saturated fat, which is why a switch from red meat to white meat does not lower cholesterol levels very well. Foods from plants let you avoid all the cholesterol and nearly all the saturated fat.

How to Read Your Cholesterol Test

A doctor measuring your cholesterol level is actually checking several different values. Here is what the numbers actually mean (the numbers in parentheses come from the new international system):

Total cholesterol. This includes all the different types of cholesterol added together and provides a good quick check of your risk of a heart attack. If your total cholesterol is:

- 150 mg/dl (3.9 mmol/L) or less: You are at very low risk of heart disease.
- About 200 mg/dl (5.2 mmol/L): You are at average risk for North Americans.
- Above 240 mg/dl (6.2 mmol/L): You are at high risk.

High-density lipoprotein (HDL). This is sometimes called "the good cholesterol" because it is carrying cholesterol out of your body. The higher your HDL, the better. To understand your HDL level, divide it by your total cholesterol and then multiply by 100.

ANIMAL PRODUCTS VS. PLANT FOODS: NO CONTEST

	CHOLESTEROL (MG)	FAT (% OF CALORIES)
Beef brisket (lean, 4 oz)	109	29
Pork sirloin (lean, 4 oz)	105	31
Chicken breast (skinless, 4 oz)	97	23
Turkey breast (skinless, 4 oz)	79	18
Halibut (4 oz)	47	19
Chinook salmon (4 oz)	96	52
Egg (boiled)	212	61
Milk (whole, 8 oz)	33	49
Milk (2% fat, 8 oz)	18	35
Apple	0	5
Baked beans	0	4
Banana	0	4
Carrots	0	3
Lentils	0	3
Potato	0	1
Spaghetti noodles	0	4
Spinach	0	9
Sweet potato	0	1

Source: J. A. T. Pennington. *Bowes and Church's Food Values of Portions Commonly Used,* 17th ed. (Philadelphia: J. B. Lippincott, 1998).

(This shows what percentage of your total cholesterol is made up of HDL.) If the result is:

- 30 percent or more: You are at very low risk of heart problems.
- About 20 percent: You are at average risk for a North American.
- Less than 20 percent: You are at higher than average risk.

For example, let's say your total cholesterol is 200 and your HDL is 50. Dividing 50 by 200 is 0.25. Multiplying the result by

100 gives you a figure of 25 percent. Not great, but better than an average North American. Notice that it is not the absolute HDL number that matters. What counts is the comparison of HDL to your total cholesterol.

Triglycerides. These are particles of fat flowing in the bloodstream. Levels above 200 mg/dl are generally considered high.

Your doctor will also measure low-density lipoprotein (LDL) and very-low-density lipoprotein, but these numbers are not usually interpreted separately from total cholesterol, HDL, and triglycerides.

How to Put Science to Work

Here is how to plan meals to lower your cholesterol level; keep it low; and, if you have artery blockages, to have the best chance of opening them up again. Use these guidelines along with your doctor's guidance about diet or other treatments that may be appropriate for you.

1. Build your menu from these four food groups:
   - whole grains such as brown rice, whole grain pasta, bread, oatmeal, and cereal
   - legumes such as beans, peas, and lentils
   - vegetables of any variety: broccoli, carrots, cauliflower, spinach, sweet potatoes, Swiss chard, etc.
   - fruits such as apples, bananas, grapefruit, oranges, pears, strawberries, and watermelons
2. Avoid all animal products. Even chicken and fish contain fat and cholesterol, and are missing the fiber your body needs for good health. The best programs for cutting cholesterol skip these foods completely.
3. Keep vegetable oils to a minimum. While liquid vegetable oils are better than animal fats, they still contain traces of saturated fats. The tropical oils (palm, palm kernel, and coconut oils) are actually quite high in saturated fat. And steer clear of foods made with fully or partially hydrogenated oils (easily found by reading labels), which can raise your cholesterol level.
4. For complete nutrition, it is important to have a source of vitamin B_{12}, which could include any common multivitamin,

fortified soy milk or cereals, or a vitamin B$_{12}$ supplement. See chapter 2 for more information on complete nutrition.

Turning these guidelines into meals is easy. Many basic and familiar foods fit the bill, from salads and baked beans to mashed potatoes, baked potatoes, and virtually all vegetables and fruits, or try veggie lasagne, veggie chili, rice pilaf, spaghetti with tomato sauce, or a bean burrito. If you would like to take advantage of the meat substitutes that have appeared in grocery stores in recent years you'll find veggieburgers, soy hot dogs, and sandwich meats, with all the flavor of the original versions. When you choose restaurants, look for international cuisine. Italian, Chinese, Japanese, Mexican, Thai, and many others have a broad range of healthy, vegetarian choices.

Adding regular exercise to your routine is remarkably simple. The regimen used to reverse heart disease is just a half-hour walk daily, or an hour walk three times per week. If you like, you can substitute any equivalent activity: bicycling, tennis, dancing, aerobics, or anything else that gets your heart pumping. See your doctor first to make sure your heart, joints, and health in general are ready for exercise, and off you go!

Foods with Special Effects

Certain foods have unusual abilities to lower your cholesterol or to protect your heart in other ways. Don't try to use them to counter the effects of a bad diet, but they do work along with a healthy diet for added power.

- Oat products are loaded with soluble fiber, which traps cholesterol in the digestive tract and carries it out with the wastes. You'll also find soluble fiber in beans, barley, vegetables, and fruits.
- Soy products such as soy hot dogs, veggieburgers, tofu, or soy milk present two major advantages. Not only do they replace the taste and texture of animal products, usually with much less fat and no cholesterol, but they also have a special cholesterol-lowering effect.
- Garlic lowers cholesterol, too. There's no need to have an entire knob of garlic on your pasta or salad. The amount that works in research studies is just a half to one clove per day.

- Walnuts are as high in fat as any other nut, but in doses of about three ounces per day, they do lower cholesterol levels.
- Beta-carotene, vitamin E, and vitamin C protect your arteries from the damage cholesterol can cause. These natural antioxidants protect against dangerous chemical reactions within the body, including those that damage artery walls and lead to blockages.

You'll recall that beta-carotene is easy to spot. It is the orange color in carrots, sweet potatoes, and pumpkins. Green, leafy vegetables contain beta-carotene, too, although the plant's deep green coloring hides it. Vitamin E is found in whole grains, vegetables, and beans. Vitamin C is in citrus fruits, of course, but also in many other fruits and vegetables such as broccoli and peppers.

If You Need Medicines

The vast majority of people with high cholesterol levels can bring them down with diet changes alone. However, some people, perhaps as many as one in ten, have a genetic tendency toward cholesterol problems. To find out whether you are in this category, follow the above diet guidelines for six to eight weeks and then check your cholesterol. If it is still high, your doctor may decide to recommend cholesterol-lowering drugs. They should always be used along with a good diet, not in place of it.

A model for combining diet and medicines comes from the research of Dr. Caldwell Esselstyn, a surgeon at the Cleveland Clinic in Cleveland, Ohio. Like other physicians, Dr. Esselstyn had been impressed by the near absence of heart disease is very poor countries where cholesterol levels were phenomenally low. So for patients struggling unsuccessfully with heart disease, he focused on getting their cholesterol levels down to where they might be had his office been in China or rural South Africa. Many had cholesterol levels hovering at 240, 260, or higher, and he aimed to get them all down below 150.

He began with a pure vegetarian (vegan) diet, throwing out anything with even a trace of animal fat or cholesterol. If cholesterol levels stubbornly remained above 150 despite the diet, Esselstyn added cholesterol-lowering drugs.

The results were dramatic. Chest pains diminished, then stopped. Nearly everyone lost weight and gained energy. After five years on the program, patients whose life expectancy had been measured in months were still alive. Angiograms revealed that the blockages in their arteries were reversing, meaning that the accumulated plaque was actually dissolving without surgery. It was as if his patients were becoming virtually heart-attack-proof. After twelve years, despite their having life-threatening disease at the start, all but one were alive and well, a remarkable medical achievement.

Hormone Replacement: The Experiment That Failed

Hormone replacement is not the way to cut the risk for heart disease. As we saw in chapter 5, large studies have disproved the once widely held notion that estrogen by prescription protects the heart. Although initial studies seemed promising, a large trial funded by Wyeth-Ayerst, the manufacturer of Premarin, the most widely used estrogen brand, proved otherwise. Over a four-year period, women taking Premarin had as many heart attacks and heart-related deaths as women taking a placebo—and, if anything, they had them slightly earlier. The studies also called attention to the drug's link to blood clots and gallbladder disease. The bottom line: Don't look to HRT to prevent heart attacks.

Stroke

If a friend or a family member has ever had a stroke, you know it can be devastating. A stroke means that part of the brain has died after losing its normal blood supply. Sometimes this is caused by a blockage in an artery leading to the brain. In another case, called a hemorrhagic strokes, an artery has burst, and blood has flooded into the brain tissue.

The part of the brain that is damaged determines the functions that are lost. If the language centers are damaged, speech becomes difficult or impossible. When the cells that control movement are killed off, paralysis results. When the network of neurons used in reasoning is damaged, the result is dementia, which can be mild or severe.

Recent studies give clear evidence about means of avoiding strokes. The key steps—a vegetarian diet, regular exercise, and not smoking—prevent strokes in much the same way that they prevent heart attacks. They help you steer clear of artery blockages that could stop normal blood flow to your brain, and keep your blood pressure low to help prevent breaks in blood vessels.

A little moderate exercise is more powerful than many realize. As part of the Nurses' Health Study, 72,488 female nurses aged forty to sixty-five were followed from 1986, completing detailed physical activity questionnaires three times during the study. The most physically active women had only *half* the stroke risk of the least active ones.

Playing sports, going to the gym, or simply walking all proved effective for reducing risk. Of course, the longer and brisker the walks, the more protection they provided. This particular study showed that for every hour spent in moderate to vigorous physical activity each week, stroke risk was cut by roughly 10 percent— even for those women who had previously been inactive.

And steer clear of diets that discourage you from eating hearty breads. The Harvard Nurses' Health Study also evaluated the diets of 75,521 U.S. women, aged thirty-eight to sixty-three, for twelve years, asking them to complete detailed questionnaires about the foods they ate. Risk of stroke was 31 percent higher for those eating the least whole grain foods compared to those eating the most, after adjusting for smoking activity level, age, and other factors. Incorporating exercise with a healthy diet, and kicking the smoking habit for good, provided the greatest degree of protection.

Whole grain foods included dark breads, whole grain breakfast cereals, popcorn, oatmeal, wheat germ, brown rice, bran, and other grains such as bulgur, kasha, and couscous. They proved effective against ischemic stroke, the kind caused by narrowed blood vessels.

Your body is built to last a century or more. While your heart and blood vessels have a big job to do, healthy foods and regular exercise will help them stay strong and healthy.

9

Using Foods to
Fight Arthritis

Most of us take for granted that we'll stay strong and healthy, able to do whatever we'd like for years to come. But when arthritis enters our lives, even the slightest movement becomes painful, sometimes impossible. It hurts to shake hands. It's hard to open a jar or write with a pen, and it feels like we are on a one-way street to the infirmities of old age.

If joint pain has slowed you down, you'll want to look at the latest from the world of nutrition. Research shows that for a surprising number of people, a few simple diet changes can make joint problems improve—or even disappear altogether. The disease comes in a great many forms, so let's start with a look at what kind of arthritis you have. Here are the most common types:

Rheumatoid arthritis. This causes joint pain and stiffness, usually starting in the hands or the feet. Sometimes the pain spreads to the shoulders, elbows, hips, knees, ankles, and neck. It is an autoimmune disease, meaning that your white blood cells—which are supposed to be fighting against bacteria, viruses, and cancer cells—have begun to attack *you.* Specifically, they are attacking the tender synovial membranes that line the inside of each joint. As time goes on, this attack damages and deforms the entire joint. For reasons that no one has yet figured out, rheumatoid arthritis affects women about three times more often than men.

Osteoarthritis. This is also called degenerative joint disease and can be thought of as wear and tear on the cartilage that cushions the ends of the bones inside the joints. As cartilage wears away, the bones start to rub against each other, causing pain and making movement difficult. It is very common in older people—ten times more common than rheumatoid arthritis—and usually shows up in the hands and the weight-bearing joints—the hips, knees, feet, and the back. If you have arthritis in the finger joints closest to your nails, it is probably osteoarthritis rather than rheumatoid.

Gout. This occurs when crystals of uric acid form in the joints, sparking inflammation and pain. It comes in acute attacks, usually starting in the big toe and spreading to other joints. Unlike rheumatoid and osteoarthritis, gout strikes more often in men.

Ankylosing spondylitis. This is a form of arthritis in the spine. It leads to stiffness in the lower back and eventually to damage to the vertebral joints. It occurs most often in young men.

In this chapter we will look at how foods can ease your joints, focusing especially on rheumatoid arthritis, where diet changes have brought remarkable results for many people. If you have osteoarthritis or ankylosing spondylitis, please review this section as well, because the same diet changes that often work for rheumatoid arthritis may be helpful to you, too. Then we will look at the important role foods play in gout.

Foods Emerge as a Cause—and a Cure

Over the past two decades, researchers have slowly but surely nailed down evidence that foods play an important role in rheumatoid arthritis and other forms of the disease. First came surprising reports of individuals who were essentially cured after making rather minor adjustments in their diets.

In 1981 the *British Medical Journal* reported the case of a woman who had suffered with rheumatoid arthritis for twenty-five years before discovering that her symptoms were caused by corn.

When she carefully avoided corn products, her arthritis simply went away. Several weeks after this remarkable recovery, however, her pain and stiffness returned. It began to look as if her improvement was simply temporary—nothing more than a placebo effect of the diet change. But, as the journal report recounted, researchers then found out that her cook had started using cornstarch as a thickener. When it was removed from the diet, her symptoms again vanished.

At about the same time, another research team published the case of an eight-year-old girl with juvenile arthritis that turned out to be caused by dairy products. Even the traces of milk in a chocolate bar were enough to spark pain and stiffness in her hands, wrists, feet, hips, and knees. The disease became so severe that she had to be hospitalized nine times. Her doctors and family were skeptical at first that something as seemingly innocent as cow's milk could trigger such a serious case of arthritis. But in repeated tests it became clear that avoiding dairy products cured her joint pains, while returning them to her diet meant pain was sure to follow.

Many doctors have been slow to accept the diet-arthritis link, despite the fact that they have had little else to offer arthritis sufferers. After all, typical arthritis medicines only relieve pain and stiffness temporarily, doing nothing to stop the progressive joint damage, and many second-line arthritis drugs have major side effects. Recently, however, the scientific evidence has become too strong to ignore. Perhaps most decisive was a carefully executed research study published in *Lancet,* a prominent British medical journal. The researchers examined twenty-six arthritis patients and documented their symptoms in detail. They then asked them to eliminate certain foods (for a list, see below). The results were quick and impressive. Pain and stiffness melted away, and grip strength returned. It was as if the patients had found a powerful new drug that eased their joints, yet the "drug" was simply a change in diet. The research team checked the patients a year later and found that their improvements were continuing.

Not everyone can blame their symptoms on food, but if diet changes go far enough, as many as 60 percent of people get better and, for some, arthritis goes away completely.

Feeling Young Again

Nancy, a forty-three-year-old pharmacist, had been suffering with rheumatoid arthritis since she was twenty years old. She had tried many different medications and eventually needed joint surgery. But her arthritis continued to worsen and, by the time she was forty, the pain had become excruciating. Walking was increasingly difficult, and she felt she was on an ever-shrinking tether. From a new doctor, she learned that dairy products and eggs could be arthritis triggers, and she decided to see how she felt without them. The results were dramatic. Within a month she was totally pain-free. Her grip strength improved, and she felt ten years younger. For her, a diet change proved more powerful than all the arthritis drugs put together.

Foods That Trigger Arthritis

These foods have been commonly found in research studies to trigger arthritis symptoms:

dairy products	citrus fruits
corn	potatoes
meats	tomatoes
wheat, oats, rye	nuts and peanuts
eggs	coffee

Dairy products are the most common trigger, as is also true for migraines (see chapter 11). This means *all* dairy products, including skim or whole cow's milk, goat's milk, cheese, yogurt, etc. Similarly, the meat category includes *all* meats: beef, pork, chicken, turkey, fish, etc. While this list applies principally to rheumatoid arthritis, people with other forms of the disease sometimes benefit from eliminating these triggers, too.

To find out which food (or foods) is bothering you, simply avoid these ten foods for about three weeks to let your joints cool down. In their place, have generous amounts of these "pain safe" foods, which do not contribute to joint problems:

- brown rice
- fruits: apricots, cranberries, pears, prunes, etc. (avoid citrus fruits, bananas, peaches, or tomatoes)
- cooked green, yellow, and orange vegetables: asparagus, broccoli, chard, collards, lettuce, spinach, squash, string beans, sweet potatoes, etc. (some people react to raw varieties)
- water: plain or carbonated
- condiments: salt, vinegar, maple syrup, and vanilla extract

In the back of this book you'll find many recipes that are free of trigger foods. After three weeks, if your symptoms have improved, reintroduce the trigger foods into your diet one at a time, every two days. Have a generous amount of the food you are testing, so you can tell how it affects you. If your joints flare up again, eliminate the offending food, and let your joints cool down again before bringing in another food item.

If you would like extra power against arthritis, you should know that medically supervised fasting has shown remarkable results for many people. Whether its value comes from the fact that fasting eliminates all diet triggers (along with all other foods) or from

She's Not Just Walking, She's Dancing

Shelly was a thirty-nine-year-old mother of three active daughters. She had been diagnosed with osteoarthritis at age twelve. In her late thirties, the disease became particularly acute. Her knees and hips hurt more and more, and she got to the point where she could no longer walk her dog. As she became more and more inactive, she started to gain weight, and she slipped into a depression.

When she heard that a diet adjustment might help, she felt annoyed at the need to change yet another part of her life. But she finally decided it was worth a try and started by eliminating dairy products—and that hit the nail on the head. The change surprised everyone in her family. Within three days, she felt better. Her pain went away, she regained her ability to walk normally, and she even danced at her brother's wedding. She felt that she had suddenly gotten her life back.

some other biochemical response to fasting is not yet clear. The vast majority of patients improve, often dramatically.

Natural Oils

Remember the Tin Man in *The Wizard of Oz?* He stood with frozen joints until Dorothy loosened him up with a drop or two of oil. Surprising as it may sound, certain natural food oils act like gentle medicines, easing your joints and giving you extra power against arthritis. Don't even think about them, though, if you haven't first checked for food triggers. If, for example, your arthritis is triggered by milk products, it is much more effective to eliminate them than to try to counteract their effects by adding oils—or medications, for that matter.

How do these oils work? They fight inflammation—which is your body's natural reaction to injury. You'll see it every time you burn your finger or scrape your elbow. The injured area gradually swells, turns red, and becomes warm to the touch as increasing blood flow brings in germ-fighting white blood cells and healing nutrients. As we saw earlier, the problem in rheumatoid arthritis is that the white blood cells' battle has mistakenly turned against your joint linings. Instead of killing bacteria, your white blood cell soldiers end up attacking your own tissues.

Simple painkillers such as aspirin or ibuprofen work by blocking inflammation. Natural oils do essentially the same thing, without side effects. There are two you should know about:

Gamma-linolenic acid (GLA). This is found in borage oil, evening primrose oil, blackcurrant oil, and hemp oil. Researchers at the University of Pennsylvania and elsewhere have found that these oils reduce swelling, tenderness, pain, and stiffness.

GLA-rich natural oils include the following:

Blackcurrant oil	17–18%
Borage oil	24%
Evening primrose oil	8–10%
Hemp oil	19%

Borage oil has the highest GLA content (¼ teaspoon supplies 300 milligrams of GLA), meaning it gives you the most benefit for the least amount of oil. You'll find GLA-rich oils at any health food store, or you can order them from the same source that supplies research teams, a company called Health From the Sun in Sunapee, New Hampshire (800-447-2229).

Alpha-linolenic acid (ALA). This is found in flaxseed oil, and to a lesser extent in canola, wheat germ, walnut, and several other oils. There are also traces of ALA in many vegetables, beans, and fruits. ALA is in the omega-3 family of fats, the group that also includes fish oils. However, you can skip fish and the chemical contaminants they harbor by using flax oil instead.

Natural ALA-rich oils include the following:

Canola oil	11%
Flaxseed oil	53–62%
Linseed oil	53%
Soybean oil	7%
Walnut oil	10%
Wheat germ oil	7%

If your diet is rich in vegetables and beans, traces of ALA will end up on your plate naturally, although not nearly as much as you'll find in flaxseed oil. Green leafy vegetables such as purslane, lettuce, broccoli, spinach, and kale contain significant amounts of ALA, as do navy, pinto, or lima beans, and peas and split peas. Citrus fruits contain ALA, but be careful with them until you are sure they are not pain triggers for you.

On the other hand, if your diet is loaded with meats, dairy products, shortenings, and cooking oils (e.g., corn oil or cottonseed oil), their unfriendly fats get packed into your cells, crowding out the ALA you need. If a doctor were to remove a small fat sample from your thigh and send it to a laboratory, he or she could tell a lot about what you have been eating lately. Chicken fat, fish fat, beef fat, and fryer grease get packed into the membranes of your cells and stay there until other fats push them out. If you were eating lots of vegetables, fruits, and beans, you would likely have little body fat overall, but the fat you did have would be high in healthy ALA and the other omega-3s that are made from it. People on meaty, greasy diets pack these unhealthy fats into their cells and have weaker defenses against inflammation.

To use natural oils against arthritis, include each of the following every day, usually with the evening meal:

1. Borage, blackcurrant, or evening primrose oil, containing 1.4 grams of GLA
2. Flaxseed oil, one tablespoon (or four capsules)
3. Vitamin E, 400 IU. If you have high blood pressure, limit the dose to 100 IU, because vitamin E can reduce your blood-clotting ability.

Allow several weeks to see their full effects. If oils cause loose stools, reduce your dose. Like all supplements, you should use them in consultation with your doctor, and avoid them if you are or may be pregnant. GLA may increase the possibility of miscarriage.

More Power for Healthy Joints

Would you like more power against arthritis? There are other gentle and natural approaches to arthritis you should know about.

Ginger. This has been used for centuries in traditional Indian ayurvedic medicine as an arthritis treatment. Modern science has shown how it works: Ginger blocks the enzymes that spark inflammation. A research team in Denmark reported remarkable results with ginger in twenty-eight patients with rheumatoid arthritis and eighteen with osteoarthritis. The usual dose is $\frac{1}{2}$ to 1 teaspoon (1 to 2 grams) of powdered ginger each day, mixed into water or added to food. Allow four to twelve weeks for benefits to appear.

Capsaicin. Pronounced "cap say' a sin," this is an extract from hot peppers and is sold in drugstores as a cream under the brand names Dolorac and Zostrix, among others. You simply apply it to sore joints twice a day. At first it tingles a bit, but as you continue to use it, the tingling diminishes and joint pain abates. It works by depleting a chemical called substance P that nerves use to transmit pain signals.

Vitamin E. This reduces the pain and stiffness of osteoarthritis, even when used without GLA or ALA. The usual dose is 400 IU each day, or 100 IU if you have high blood pressure.

Weight loss. This is important in preventing and treating osteoarthritis. Researchers have found that every ten pounds of excess weight increase the risk of osteoarthritis in the knees by 30 percent. It is not just that extra weight strains your joints—the joint problems can even show up in your hands. Researchers suspect that body fat works its mischief by producing estrogens, and that these hormones make arthritis more likely. Indeed, women with arthritis often have other signs of excess estrogen, such as uterine fibroids. The healthiest and most effective way to lose weight is to focus on changing the type of food you eat, rather than trying to meet a strict calorie limit. For details see chapter 6.

Check your iron level. You need a small amount of iron in your diet for your red blood cells to carry oxygen. But in excess, iron contributes to joint damage by encouraging the formation of free radicals, unstable molecules that can attack your body tissues. As we have seen, the meat-based diets that are common in Western countries are so high in iron that they push many of us into a mild form of iron overload, especially after menopause. Do you have too much iron stored in your body? To check, ask your doctor for these simple tests (also described in chapter 1):

1. Serum ferritin (normal values are 12-200 mcg/l)
2. Serum iron and total iron binding capacity (TIBC). When the serum iron measurement is divided by TIBC, the result should be 16 to 50 percent for women and 16 to 62 percent for men.

If these tests show you have excess iron in your blood, you can gradually bring your iron level back to normal with regular exercise and, as we learned in chapter 1, by donating blood. This altruistic act gives a person in need the extra iron you are anxious to be rid of.

To help keep your iron level in the normal range, get your iron from whole grains, beans, vegetables, and fruits in your diet, rather than from meats. Plants contain iron in a form your body can easily regulate. Heme iron, found in meats, bombards your body with iron that is difficult to get rid of.

Antibiotics against Arthritis?

Antibiotics have emerged as an important, although controversial, treatment for arthritis. Certain bacterial infections—salmonella, campylobacter, or yersinia, which are common contaminants in raw chicken and beef—are well-known causes of joint pain that can linger on long after the initial gastrointestinal illness they often cause is gone. Researchers suspect that other bacteria also are involved in many cases of arthritis. A great resource on antibiotic treatments for arthritis is Dr. Gabe Mirkin, a nationally known progressive physician (800-986-4754, www.DrMirkin.com) Ask your doctor whether antibiotics might help in your case.

Diet Changes for Gout

If you have gout, you will likely need medicines, perhaps even hospitalization. But you should also look at two parts of your diet that can increase the risk of gout. Meats, especially shellfish, sardines, anchovies, and organ meats (e.g., liver and kidneys), and alcohol, especially beer, encourage uric acid to deposit in your joints, causing the misery of gout. Steer clear of these foods and build your diet from vegetables, grains, and fruits. Be sure to stay on your medications during the transition, however, since gout sometimes strikes during times of dietary change.

Joint pains can make life miserable. But a great many people have gotten surprising relief from simple adjustments in their eating habits—and all the side effects are good ones. A diet rich in vegetables, fruits, beans, and whole grains will help you lose weight, cut your cholesterol, and build your energy. Steering clear of trigger foods, and adding supplements if you want them, can make a world of difference.

10

Keeping Bones Strong

Osteoporosis has been called the "silent disease," deteriorating bones often without warning signs, leaving many older women incapacitated with fractures, in pain, and with significant medical bills. Throughout recent years, physicians and nutritionists have recommended high doses of calcium—mainly through dairy products and supplements—as the primary means of prevention. The U.S. government, in its dietary guidelines, strongly advocates milk drinking. Dozens of celebrities have even joined the promotion, sporting "milk mustaches" in a high-dollar ad campaign urging everyone to drink up, yet the risk for osteoporosis and related bone breaks is *not* decreasing.

Ten million Americans, 80 percent of whom are women, already have the disease, characterized as porous, brittle bones. The National Osteoporosis Foundation estimates that 10 million more individuals are at risk due to low bone mass. One in two U.S. women will have an osteoporosis-related bone fracture in her lifetime. Why is this happening in countries where dairy consumption is so high?

The largest study assessing the benefits of calcium for preventing osteoporosis revealed the futility of relying on dairy products to protect bones. The Harvard Nurses' Health Study followed 77,761 women aged thirty-four to fifty-nine, over a twelve-year period and found that those who drank three or more glasses of milk per day had no reduction in the risk of hip or arm fractures, compared to those who drank little or no milk. In fact, milk drinkers' fracture rates were slightly *higher.* Clearly there are other factors at work here.

Very different from the messages we hear in the media, calcium researchers have continually found that countries with the highest calcium intakes actually have higher, not lower, rates of osteoporosis. The reason may lie in other concomitant dietary characteristics. Where calcium intakes are highest, large dairy industries exist, producing not only large quantities of milk, cheese, yogurt, and butter, but also meat from dairy cattle whose milk production has declined. Where meat consumption is greatest, osteoporosis rates are high. Researchers, and some physicians, now understand the link: excess protein causes calcium *loss.* There was a time when we knew of no real detriments to loading up on protein. In fact, we thought family dinners had to center around a big steak, chicken, or pork. Now that misinformation has come back to hurt us.

Researchers have found that physical activity is vitally important to proper bone development, too. A study of young women found that bone density was significantly affected by how much exercise the girls got in their teen years, the time when girls develop 40 to 50 percent of their skeletal mass. Calcium intake, on the other hand, made no difference. The Penn State researchers focused on hip bone density, a common site for fractures in women with osteoporosis. For six years, eighty-one twelve-year-old girls were evaluated with respect to dietary habits and sports activities while taking part in a calcium supplementation study. Consistent with past studies, intake of calcium above 900 milligrams per day (two glasses of milk) had no lasting effect on bone strength, but regular exercise did. Researchers remind us that while serious athletics and team sports are fine for some, bone-strengthening benefits come simply from walking for thirty minutes each day. Added benefit will be achieved by including regular weight-bearing exercises such as backpacking or walking with hand weights. Don't let group weight-lifting classes scare you away. Visit your local gym and you're likely to find these classes full of women. You can start with three-pound weights and, in no time, brand-new muscle groups will have you lifting more and more.

Excess Protein Spells Trouble for Bones

A group of Yale researchers looked at hip fracture rates in sixteen different countries, focusing on women over fifty because osteoporosis is particularly aggressive in women after menopause. They found that countries with a high calcium intake happened to be those where Western diets—high in meat and dairy products—were popular. A closer look at meat consumption in these populations revealed that, indeed, the more meat people ate, the more fractures they had.

When researchers feed animal protein to volunteers and test their urine, they find it loaded with calcium. Here's why: When protein is digested, its component amino acids come apart and pass into the blood, making the blood slightly acidic. However, the body is extremely finicky about how acidic the blood gets because even a tiny change in acid levels can derange body chemistry. In the process of neutralizing that acidity, calcium is pulled from the bones and ends up being lost in the urine. A report in the *American Journal of Clinical Nutrition* showed that when research subjects eliminated meats, cheese, and eggs from their diet, they cut their calcium losses in half.

The bone-dissolving effects of America's meat- and cheese-heavy diet was recently illustrated in a large study from the University of California at San Francisco (UCSF). Researchers divided more than nine thousand women, sixty-five and older, into five groups and found the women who consumed the most acidic foods (protein-rich meats and cheeses) had 3.7 times more hip fractures than those eating the least acidic foods.

Another UCSF scientist studied diet and hip fracture rates in thirty-three countries, reporting that differences in ratio of plant to animal food accounted for 70 percent of the variation in fracture rates. The best bone-protecting diet is rich in fruits and vegetables, which are high in potassium. While dairy products do contain calcium, the acid they provide, especially from hard cheeses, adds to bone deterioration. Low-fat, calcium-rich beans, green vegetables, and fortified juices provide calcium and ensure it stays where it belongs.

Limit Caffeine and Salt

Caffeine and salt in the diet pose problems as well. Caffeine, acting as a mild diuretic, causes calcium loss via the kidneys. For post-menopausal women, the effects of calcium loss through soda, coffee, and tea drinking is significant. The same is true of salt. For an average person, cutting sodium in half reduces the daily calcium requirement by about 160 milligrams. Again, it is the body's need to regulate levels of sodium, just as it regulates protein. When there is too much sodium, the kidneys try to get rid of it, taking calcium along as well. Natural foods from plants, which are high in potassium rather than sodium, have the opposite effect. They help keep calcium in the bones, apparently by reducing calcium loss from the kidneys.

Another Reason to Quit Smoking

Another risk for osteoporosis is smoking. Australian researchers studied forty-one sets of identical twins, all of whom were adult women. They found that if one twin smoked and the other did not, the smoker's bones were about 10 percent less dense in the spine and about 5 percent less dense in the hip and thigh bones, even though their genes were, of course, the same. This difference can mean a 44 percent increase in the risk of hip fracture.

Vegetarian Bone Builders

The healthiest, most absorbable sources of calcium are found in green, leafy vegetables such as broccoli, which contains 115 milligrams per 100-gram serving. An exception is spinach, which is different from other greens because it has a less-absorbable form of calcium. Beans, lentils, and other legumes are good sources of calcium as well as omega-3 fatty acids, cholesterol-lowering soluble fiber, and complex carbohydrates. As for supplements, the best source is found in calcium-fortified orange juice. It is more absorbable than calcium carbonate supplements.

Avoiding meat and other calcium depleters makes it much easier to get, and keep, 400 to 500 milligrams—as recommended by the World Health Organization—in the body each day. Besides substantial protein, meats (including poultry) also contain phosphorus in amounts fifteen times greater than the calcium they provide. The tremendous phosphorous overload encourages calcium loss. You'll want to avoid overdoing soda consumption as well. Their phosphoric acid and caffeine combination swiftly move calcium out via the kidneys.

Swapping meats and other animal products for fruits, vegetables, legumes, and nuts provides added defense from the mineral boron, which also helps keep calcium in the bones.

Get a Little Sunlight

A little sunlight and daily exercise are important in preventing osteoporosis, too. Bones respond to the push and pull of exercise, especially the weight-bearing variety, by becoming stronger and denser. The effect is really remarkable. Take studies done on athletes, for example. Tennis players have significantly greater bone density in the arm they grip their racket with, compared to their less-active arm. Brief periods of time in the sun turn on the body's natural production of vitamin D, helping the digestive tract to absorb calcium from foods. Vitamin D is also stored in body fat and muscle, accumulating plenty for rainy days.

False Hope in Hormone Replacement Therapy

It has become common practice for physicians to prescribe HRT for their female patients after menopause, but this hasn't provided the protection many—especially its manufacturers—hoped it would. Researchers have found that even if postmenopausal women take estrogens faithfully, most will still lose bone, albeit at a slower rate. And as they approach their seventies and eighties, the effects of estrogen replacement wane, and many women have fractures in spite of hormone use. As we saw in chapter 7, taking HRT increases your risk for gallbladder disease and breast and uterine cancer, frightening prospects, particularly when we know so much about safer approaches, such as the positive effects of vegetable foods on bone strength.

Women on low-fat, plant-based diets have lower levels of estrogen in their blood before menopause, are adapted to those levels, and have less of a change at menopause. Instead of a major dip in hormone level, they get more of a gentle readjustment. This is probably one of the major reasons why doctors in Asia report that menopausal symptoms and hip fractures are much rarer than in the West and why vegetarian women going into menopause are more likely to keep strong bones.

Rebuilding Bones

Natural progesterone, derived from various plants, most notably wild yams and soybeans, has proved to be a very beneficial treatment option for postmenopausal women, not only in slowing bone loss but also in building bone. One study showed an average bone density increase of 15 percent in a group of a hundred postmenopausal women. And, unlike estrogens, progesterone does not appear to increase cancer risk. Progesterone often reduces hot flashes, eases fibrocystic breast pain, improves thyroid functioning, and encourages weight loss. Despite these profound benefits, progesterone remains overshadowed by heavily marketed prescription drug therapies. As a natural compound it cannot be patented by drug companies, leaving them little financial incentive to market or sell it.

On a Western diet, heavy with animal protein, phosphorus, sodium, and caffeine, and aggravated by smoking and inactivity, osteoporosis will continue to be a major health problem. Simply adding extra calcium or hormone preparations to this mix has proved an ineffective defense. Physicians could be making great strides in reducing osteoporosis if they discussed the vitally important research findings described in this chapter with their female patients, especially when they are still young.

Prevention *is* possible, through a diet based on wholesome foods plus daily activity and a few minutes of rejuvenating sunlight.

11

Free Yourself from Headaches

When headaches strike, most of us reach for a bottle of pain relievers. But a powerful new approach lets you get to their cause. The key may not be in your medicine cabinet but on your plate. For years many migraine sufferers have suspected that certain foods—especially red wine, cheese, and chocolate—can trigger their headaches. Doctors remained skeptical until researchers at London's Hospital for Sick Children proved the food-headache link. They carefully eliminated suspected trigger foods from the diets of eighty-eight children suffering from frequent migraines. In days, seventy-eight of the children were cured, four were improved, and only six got no benefit from the menu change.

First let's look at *your* headaches. The treatment that is right for one kind of headache can be entirely different from that for another. Here's an example.

A young woman had dull, steady headaches virtually every afternoon. They started at her temples and passed through her head like a knife. At the time she was working at a large law firm. Her hours were long, and her workload kept growing. Her husband, also a lawyer, worked long hours, too. Their three-year-old son, who was in day care, often needed extra attention for a sore throat or a fever. For some reason it always fell to her to deal with these emergencies. At first two aspirin knocked her headaches out, but as time went on they became more and more resistant to painkillers. She went to her doctor to see if she was having migraines.

Can you make the diagnosis? Look at the following descriptions of headache types.

Migraines. These are not just bad headaches. They have a characteristic pattern, usually involving just one side of your head, and the pain is throbbing, rather than a dull, constant ache. Along with the pain come nausea, vomiting, and sensitivity to light and sounds. Some people have a brief warning aura of flashing lights or visual distortions before the headache arrives. A migraine is not fleeting. You can suffer for hours, sometimes days. Neurologists believe that a constriction of blood vessels in the brain causes the peculiar visual effects. Then blood vessels expand, causing throbbing pain. Migraines can be triggered not only by foods but also by stress, weather changes, perfume, cigarette smoke, sunlight, too much sleep, or too little sleep. Once a migraine has arrived, falling asleep will often make it go away.

Tension headaches. These do not throb or pulse the way a migraine does. It is a diffuse, constant ache that is believed to be caused by tension in the muscles under the scalp. The headache arrives during times of stress.

Cluster headaches. These are excruciating, centering around one eye, which turns red and begins to water. It is much briefer than a migraine, lasting only an hour or so, and does not include the nausea, vomiting, light sensitivity, or visual aura that migraines often have. Its name refers to the fact that the headaches come in clusters, arriving day after day on the same side of your head, and then vanish for long periods.

Sinus headaches. These hit you in the forehead or under your eyes as a constant ache, rather than a throbbing pain. Environmental or food allergies are often to blame.

Caffeine withdrawal headaches. These are no great mystery. The dull, constant ache kicks in when coffee drinkers miss their morning cup of coffee.

Temporal Arteritis. This is caused by an inflamed artery that is firm to the touch and very sensitive, causing a throbbing headache on one side. It is often accompanied by fatigue and aching muscles and joints. A blood test, called a sedimentation rate, is often abnormally high in temporal arteritis. Doctors prescribe steroids to prevent serious complications, including blindness.

Blood vessel abnormalities. These can cause headaches that occur repeatedly on one side of the head. While migraines will at least occasionally affect either side of your head and cluster headaches may switch sides when a new cluster begins, headaches caused by an abnormal blood vessel stay on the same side and often cause nerve symptoms.

Glaucoma. This is increased pressure within the eye and can cause a headache with eye pain and vomiting.

So what kind of headache did the young lawyer have? As you have no doubt figured out by now, she did not have migraines. Migraines are throbbing, one-sided headaches, while her pain was a constant ache brought on during times of stress. Most likely she was suffering from tension headaches—by far the most common type.

Knock Out Your Migraines

Sometimes medicines make a world of difference when you are suffering from migraines. But drugs can lose their effectiveness,

See Your Doctor

There are many headache causes, and it is important to see your doctor for a diagnosis, especially if headaches are new for you, are severe or persistent, or are accompanied by any of the following:

- back or neck pain
- fever
- a change in nerve function, strength, coordination, or senses
- a run-down feeling with muscle or joint pain
- drowsiness or difficulty concentrating

and overuse suppresses your natural painkilling endorphins, leading to more and more frequent headaches. If you have migraines, it pays to look for what might be causing them. A menu change is often the answer.

While the Hospital for Sick Children study mentioned earlier was among the first to nail down specific food triggers, researchers have long speculated about links between diet and migraines. In 1778 John Fothergill wrote that the "sick headache" comes "from inattention to diet, either in respect to kind or quantity or both. . . ." The culprits, he wrote, were "milk and butter, fat meats and spices, especially common black pepper and meat pies and rich baked puddings."

Recent scientific studies have pinpointed the causes much more accurately. For children, foods play a role in the vast majority of migraines. For adults, diet is a major contributor in 20 to 50 percent of cases. Often more than one food plays a role.

Twelve foods—the "dirty dozen"—are especially common migraine triggers:

dairy products	nuts and peanuts
chocolate	tomatoes
eggs	onions
citrus fruits	corn
meat	apples
wheat (bread, pasta, etc.)	bananas

As you look at this list, it is important to know that you are not sensitive to all twelve triggers. It may be that only one or two apply to you. Here is how to identify *your* triggers: For ten days, remove all of the "dirty dozen" foods from your diet. This is more than enough time for your headaches to stop coming. Then reintroduce these foods, one at a time. Starting at the bottom of the list, bring in one food every two days, having a generous amount so you can see how it affects you. If you get a headache, eliminate that food again. If not, you can keep it in your diet. Begin the test with bananas, having several bananas a day for two days. Then move on to apples, then corn, etc.

You may be wondering why foods as healthful as citrus fruits, apples, or bananas could trigger headaches. Well, just as you may have known people who get a rash from strawberries—and there is nothing unhealthy about strawberries—many foods can cause reactions if you are sensitive to them. Migraines are apparently a reaction to proteins in the food.

Note that dairy products are the most common triggers. Many people consume milk in a mistaken attempt to protect their bones (see chapter 11), or are hooked on cheese or ice cream. Avoiding these products can help enormously. Switching to nonfat varieties does not help: The problem is not the dairy fat, but the dairy proteins. Happily, now that soy milk and rice milk are widely available, eliminating cow's milk is easy.

Wheat is also a common trigger. This doesn't mean you have to swear off breads or pasta. You'll find wheat-free versions made from rice, millet, quinoa, and other grains at health food stores.

Certain beverages can cause migraines, too. Red wine is the best-known culprit, but migraines can be triggered by other alcoholic beverages and by sodas flavored with aspartame (NutraSweet). Instead of sodas, try sparkling water or mineral water.

Coffee drinkers tend to have more headaches than other people, especially when they miss their morning cup. Ironically, however, coffee also can be a migraine treatment. If you take one to two cups of strong coffee just as a migraine is beginning, the flood of caffeine can actually knock out the headache. Caffeine is a natural blood vessel constrictor, which is why it is often added to over-the-counter headache remedies. Once you are habituated to coffee, tea, sodas, chocolate bars, or other caffeinated products, missing them for a day can make you feel out of sorts and bring on headaches.

Some food additives can trigger migraines. Especially common offenders include monosodium glutamate (MSG) and nitrites, which are used to cure bacon, hot dogs, and other luncheon meats. MSG is used as a flavor enhancer, especially in Chinese food. If you are sensitive to MSG, you'll feel tightness around your face about twenty minutes after the meal begins. Ask the waiter to leave out the MSG.

Pain-Safe Foods

Certain foods are "pain safe," meaning they virtually never contribute to headaches. If you have migraines, you would do well to include them in your diet in generous amounts, especially during an elimination diet. They include:

- rice, especially brown rice
- cooked green, orange, and yellow vegetables
- cooked or dried fruits other than citrus fruits, apples, bananas, peaches, or tomatoes
- water
- condiments: salt, vinegar, maple syrup, and vanilla extract

If the food elimination test did not identify trigger foods for you, it may be that some other, less common trigger food is causing your headaches. The way to test this is to build your menu *entirely* from pain-safe foods for ten days or so. If your headaches disappear, you can then reintroduce your normal foods one at a time to see which one (or ones) trigger your headaches.

Normally, food triggers do their mischief quickly, causing headaches within a few hours. Sometimes, however, you may have to include a food in your routine for a few days before the headaches start. Also, you may find you are more sensitive to migraine triggers the week before your period. Sadly, the culprits are often foods you are fond of.

Three of the "dirty dozen" foods are best left off your plate permanently: meats, dairy products, and eggs. They have enough cholesterol, fat, and animal proteins to contribute to serious health concerns. Moreover, their load of fat and lack of fiber can disturb your natural hormone balance, which contributes to migraines, as we will see below.

What Is It about Chocolate, Cheese, and Red Wine?

Many migraine sufferers feel much better when they steer clear of chocolate, cheese, and alcohol, especially red wine. What is it about these foods that causes such a problem? Chocolate contains an amphetaminelike chemical called phenylethylamine (PEA), which alters blood flow within the brain. Certain sensitizing proteins in chocolate also may be to blame. Red wine contains PEA, too, along with a huge amount of histamine, a chemical that causes the runny nose and sneezing that come with allergies. Histamine alters blood flow to the brain, just as PEA does.

Many cheeses contain PEA and histamine, along with dairy

proteins that are among the most common triggers for food-related sensitivities, including headaches.

Natural Migraine Treatments

If eliminating food triggers doesn't completely knock out your migraines, you might try these supplements:

Feverfew. This has been used since the Middle Ages for arthritis, gynecological problems, and a variety of other health conditions, including fever, which is where its name comes from. Controlled research studies show its power against migraines. You will find it at health food stores, usually as capsules (the dose is 250 milligrams per day taken on an empty stomach) or as the plant itself, in which case you simply tear off and eat two to three leaves per day. It is used as a preventive, not a treatment.

Although feverfew appears to be quite safe, researchers have not studied its side effects over long periods. It is always prudent to avoid any medication or herbal treatment during pregnancy and lactation, except as advised by your physician. If you are on any other medicine, especially anticoagulants, ask your doctor about adding feverfew.

Ginger. This blocks *prostaglandins,* the same pain-causing chemicals targeted by aspirin and ibuprofen, and may help prevent migraines. To try it, stir ½ to 1 teaspoon (1 to 2 grams) of powdered ginger into a glass of water or have it with food each day. Or you can make a tea by boiling sliced ginger for a few minutes.

Magnesium. This helps prevent migraines. In a large research study, 80 percent of participants treated with magnesium had a reduction in migraine frequency. It is available at drugstores and health food stores. The usual dose is 200 milligrams per day of elemental magnesium. You also will find magnesium in green, leafy vegetables; dried noncitrus fruits; and whole grains such as brown rice, barley, and oats.

Balancing Your Hormones

Migraines tend to hit especially often in the week before your period, when your hormones are shifting quickly. The problem is that the amount of estrogens (female sex hormones) in your blood is dropping precipitously, sending you into a kind of "estrogen withdrawal."

Once again, foods can come to your rescue. The key, as we saw in chapter 3, is to keep your fat intake to a bare minimum throughout the month. This causes your body to make less estrogen as the weeks go by, so the drop at the end of the month will be less pronounced. Fiber-rich foods help, too, because they carry excess estrogens out of your body, helping to prevent the estrogen peaks that are followed by the obligatory fall and the symptoms it can cause. Diets rich in beans, grains, and vegetables—which are naturally low in fat and high in fiber—may be why migraines are much less common in Asia and Latin America compared to the United States. The healthiest diets eliminate animal products completely and keep vegetable oils to a minimum.

Some women find relief from premenstrual headaches by combining magnesium (200 milligrams per day) with vitamin B_6 (50 to 100 milligrams per day). Avoid higher doses of vitamin B_6, which can be toxic. Normally the combination is used daily, but you also can take it for just five days before your period.

Free Yourself from Migraines

1. See your doctor. An accurate diagnosis is essential for treating headaches.
2. Track down your food triggers while having generous amounts of pain-safe foods.
3. Tame hormone changes by avoiding animal products and keeping vegetable oils to a minimum.
4. If you need more, consider feverfew, ginger, or magnesium.

Tension Headaches

Tension headaches are by far the most common type. To differentiate them from migraines, tension headaches:

- occur on both sides of the head
- are a constant, not throbbing, ache
- are mild to moderate in strength
- do not change with routine movements
- are not accompanied by nausea or light sensitivity

If you get tension headaches frequently, consider what might be contributing to them. Are you getting enough rest and exercise? Do caffeine withdrawal, hunger, or dental or sinus problems play a role?

Persistent headaches can also result from grinding your teeth as you sleep. A dentist can make a bite plate that solves this problem for many people.

For occasional headaches, pain relievers are fine. But be careful about overusing them. With chronic use they can interfere with your body's natural ability to control pain, leading to uncontrolled daily headaches. The best approach is to find a way to let tension go, especially from the muscles of your forehead or on the sides or back of your head. Try these quick tension relievers:

Neck circles. Golfer Greg Norman uses this exercise to knock out tension at stressful times. Simply lower your head to your chest, then slowly turn your head to the right, over your shoulder. Then let your head drop toward your back, then over your left shoulder, and again to the front. Do two gentle circles in each direction.

Deep breaths. The world's fastest destressor is simply to breathe in as deeply as you can. Then, before you exhale, take in a bit more air. And then take in just a bit more, really filling your lungs. Hold it for a second or two, then let it go, along with the tension in your body. This is also a good energy booster when you are fatigued.

Progressive relaxation. Close your eyes and let your breathing become slow and easy, like a person sleeping. Then, as you inhale, imagine that the air you take in travels up inside your forehead. The air collects whatever tension is there, and carries it out as you exhale. Let each breath bring relaxation in and carry tension out. Then imagine each breath carrying tension out of all the other parts of your head in succession: the sides, the back of your head, and your jaw. Each inhalation brings cool relaxation into your body, and each exhalation carries tension away. Do the same for your shoulders, arms, chest, stomach, and legs, all the way down to your feet.

If you prefer, you can tense and relax each part of your body as you go, from your head down, to help you actually feel the tension leaving each part of your body. Start by gently tensing your forehead for a moment. Then relax and let the tension go. Do the same with each part of your head, neck, and body.

Four-seven-eight breathing. Here is a simple exercise that can be done anywhere. It comes from Andrew Weil, M.D.: Open your mouth slightly, and place your tongue on the ridge behind your front teeth, keeping it there for the entire exercise. Inhale through your nose for a count of four, then hold your breath for seven counts. Now breathe out through your mouth for eight counts, making a whooshing sound as the air goes past your tongue and teeth. Do this four times. It might sound a bit silly, but try it. It works.

Rest your eyes. Lie down on your back and place a cool, damp washcloth over your eyes. Elevate your feet above the level of your heart by using a pillow or by propping them against a wall. As the cloth cools your tired eyes and the blood returns from your legs, you will feel tension leave your body.

Cluster Headaches

Cluster headaches are caused by inflammation and pressure in the veins inside the brain. Unlike tension headaches, which come on during stress, a cluster headache often begins just as you are relaxing. Along with it, one eye turns red and begins to water, and you may even find that the eyelid droops and the pupil narrows. The headache will return on the same side of your head for the entire cluster, but may switch sides if a new cluster starts later on.

There is only one clear-cut dietary trigger—alcohol—and you will want to avoid it completely during a cluster period. To track down whether other parts of your diet may contribute, you can check for the common headache trigger foods as described above for migraines. If you have cluster headaches, or any other type, it is essential to see your doctor, both for a solid diagnosis and for medical treatments if you need them.

Sinus Headaches

Sinus headaches occur especially frequently during allergy season. Pollens, dust, or other environmental irritants cause the mucous membranes in your sinuses and nasal passages to swell, leading to pressure and pain. Foods can contribute, too. The most common food allergen is dairy products. Once again, the problem is milk's protein, not its fat, so nonfat milk or yogurt is as much a problem as whole milk. Many of the other "dirty dozen" migraine triggers listed earlier also can be allergens, and can aggravate the effects of environmental allergens. It is well worth taking a break from these foods to see if your symptoms improve.

Getting Free from Headaches

You have more control over your headaches than you may have imagined. Start by visiting your doctor for an accurate diagnosis. Then check to see whether foods might be contributing to the problem. Add the easy stress busters, if you need them, to alleviate tension. And enjoy the new life that comes from breaking free of headaches.

12

Urinary Tract Health

Kidney stone. Just say the words and someone is likely to give you a grimace. No one ever forgets the suffering they experience after developing these painful pellets. The same can be true of serious bladder infections. Add in the anxiety of not knowing what is causing such discomfort and you've got a downright miserable experience. A doctor's diagnosis, and pain relief, come not a minute too soon.

Whether you've suffered a urinary tract illness yourself, or comforted a loved one at a critically painful moment, you'll be glad to know that there are simple, pain*less* steps you can take to substantially lower the risk for first-time attacks as well as recurrences. But first, some background on the little stones that cause such big problems.

Kidney stones occur when the urine becomes too concentrated, crystallizes, and forms little granules. They can remain in the body without causing pain, until they begin to move through the urinary tract. When they do, the pain (often felt in the back between the rib cage and the hip) can be excruciating. Unfortunately, kidney stones are common, affecting 5 percent of women and 10 percent of men by age seventy. Recurrence also is common, especially when the first episode occurs at a young age, has already occurred twice, or is followed by no preventive measures.

Kidney stones are most commonly made of calcium, accounting for 75 to 95 percent of cases. To form the stone, the calcium usually combines with oxalate (a part of many plant foods) and sometimes with phosphate or carbonate. Less commonly, stones form from uric acid, which is a product of protein breakdown. To keep a stone from forming in your kidney, you'll want to have less calcium, oxalate, and uric acid in your body, more water to ensure that these substances stay dissolved, and preferably both.

A Diet for Kidney Stone Prevention

It sounds simple, and it is. Drinking more water is an important step in preventing kidney stones. It dilutes the urine and keeps calcium, oxalate, and uric acid from turning into solid crystals. If you are getting about $2\frac{1}{2}$ quarts (roughly 9 cups) of liquids each day, including water, juice, soup, or other varieties, your risk for getting a kidney stone is about a third less than that of a person drinking half as much. If you are at risk, you will want to start the healthy habit of keeping fresh water with you at all times—at your desk while you work, in the cup holder as you drive, and at home in a filtering dispenser or in bottles—whichever way makes it more likely that you'll drink up. Purchasing a Thermos or other portable water bottle will add convenience. Clearer urine and more frequent urination are signs that you are on the right track.

The foods you choose are important as well. Studies have found that high-potassium foods cut the risk of kidney stones in half. So while you are increasing your daily intake of healthy, vegetarian foods—especially vegetables, fruits, and beans—for osteoporosis prevention, as discussed earlier, you'll be protected against kidney stones as well. Potassium keeps calcium in the bones and bloodstream instead of sending it out into the urine. Plant foods have a second major advantage: They are very low in sodium—another major cause for stone formation. Researchers have demonstrated that when sodium intake is cut in half, which is easy when highly processed foods are replaced with more natural, wholesome foods, your calcium requirement is reduced by about 160 milligrams. Plant foods of all varieties, including rice, potatoes, beans, oranges, bananas, cauliflower, and chickpeas, contain almost no sodium in their natural state. It's only when good foods are packed into frozen meals, cans, or other manufactured packages that large doses of salt are often added. So read labels and learn to use spices instead of salt when you cook. As you can see in the following table, plant foods are always a better choice for boosting potassium and reducing sodium in your diet.

Even though stones are often made up of calcium, there are ways to safely incorporate the mineral in your diet and keep it from causing trouble. If your physician has prescribed calcium supplements, be sure to take them with meals. Otherwise about 8 percent of it will end up in the urine, increasing the risk for stones. Taken with food, calcium binds to the oxalates in your meal, keeping them in the digestive tract. Less oxalate filtering through the kidneys means less opportunity for stones to form.

Coffee and alcoholic beverages, although not ideal for other reasons, can actually cut the risk for kidney stones. Their diuretic effect causes extra fluid to pass through the kidneys. While it causes calcium to filter along with it, you lose more water than calcium, therefore reducing risk. Of course, water is always the preferred beverage in a healthy diet.

Problem Foods for Kidney Stones

Doctors have long been advising patients with kidney disease to keep meat and all animal protein to a minimum. This is good advice for people at risk for kidney stones as well. Animal proteins overwork the kidneys and cause their filtering ability to decline.

One Harvard study found that increasing animal protein from 50 to 77 grams per day (about two extra glasses of milk) has been shown to increase stones 33 percent in men. The massive Harvard Nurses' Health Study revealed an even greater risk of stones from animal protein for women. It's not just the *amount* of protein that chicken, pork, and fish contain, it's also the *type*. These sulfur-containing amino acids pull calcium from bones and filter it through the kidneys, creating greater opportunity for stones to develop. Meats and eggs contain two to five times more of these

SODIUM AND POTASSIUM IN FOODS
(IN MILLIGRAMS)

PLANT FOODS	SODIUM	POTASSIUM
Apple (1 medium)	1	159
Banana (1 medium)	1	451
Black beans (1 cup)	1	611
Broccoli (1 cup)	44	332
Cauliflower (1 cup)	8	400
Cream of wheat (1 cup)	7	48
Grapefruit (1 medium)	0	316
Navy beans (1 cup)	2	669
Orange (1 medium)	1	250
Potato (1 medium)	16	844
Rice (1 cup)	1	60

ANIMAL PRODUCTS	SODIUM	POTASSIUM
Whole milk (1 cup)	120	370
Skim milk (1 cup)	126	406
Goat's milk (1 cup)	122	499
Human milk (1 cup)	40	128
Yogurt (1 cup)	105	351
Cheddar cheese (2 oz)	352	56
Ground beef (4 oz)	69	253
Roast beef (4 oz)	51	377
Skinless chicken breast (4 oz)	82	286
Haddock (4 oz)	98	447
Swordfish (4 oz)	130	414

amino acids than grain and beans. Needless to say, vegetarians have a great advantage. They have half the calcium loss of their meat-eating counterparts because they keep calcium in their bones, where it is needed most, and out of the kidneys, reducing the risk for stones.

Too much sugar tends to pose the same risks. Like animal protein and salt, sugar accelerates calcium loss through the kidneys. In the Nurses' Health Study, those who consumed, on average, about 60 grams or more of sugar per day had a 50 percent higher risk of stones than those who consumed only about 20 grams. You can get a better idea of your daily sugar intake by looking at the table below.

Southerners will be disappointed to learn that the risk of kidney stones is higher in warm climates. The reason, apparently, is that perspiration dehydrates the body, leading to a more concentrated urine. Also, sunlight increases the amount of vitamin D produced in the skin, which, in turn, increases the absorption of calcium from the digestive tract.

Even though many stones are made from calcium and oxalate, foods rich in oxalates, such as chocolate, nuts, and spinach, do not

SUGAR IN COMMON FOODS (IN GRAMS)

Chocolate bar (2 oz)	22–35
Cookies (3)	11–14
Corn flakes (1 cup)	2
Frosted flakes (1 cup)	17
Crackers (5)	1
Fruit cocktail (½ cup)	14
Grape jam (1 tbsp)	13
Ice cream (½ cup)	21
Soda (12 oz)	40
White bread (2 slices)	1
Marinara sauce (½ cup)	8
Ketchup (1 tbsp)	4

13

Putting It All Together

We've covered many stages in a woman's life. It's amazing how profoundly diet affects each and every one. From puberty through the childbearing years and certainly on into our mature years, food is the foundation for good health. No matter what your age today, the right diet will significantly influence your life in the coming months and years. Congratulations are in order as you turn to the recipe section of this book, putting what you have learned to work.

You'll see that unlike tricky diets that forbid carbohydrates, cost a lot of money, or require a lot of time, the perfect nutrition plan is really quite simple. That's not to say that those of you of who enjoy the culinary arts will not be able to create an elaborate and exquisite dinner party menu. You can indeed! And on busy days you'll also be able to get in and out of the kitchen in fifteen minutes, creating wonderful meals packed with antioxidants, vitamins, and minerals.

What's nice about building a diet from plant foods is that it is one plan you can share with your family, and even with friends who are lifelong dieters. Once you bring new recipes like Spicy Indian

Garbanzos and Pan-seared Portobello Mushrooms to the dinner table, you'll wonder why you ever missed out on these delicious vegetables and grains.

It is very likely that you will see changes immediately. Dwindling energy will increase, your clothes may soon fit a little more comfortably, and your mind will be free to focus on something other than calories and cholesterol. If the entire family joins in, they will benefit along with you in s , many ways. Happily, good eating habits, developed early, ofte᠆ stay with us for life. You may have been raised on overproces᠆ d convenience foods or very-high-fat hamburgers, hot dogs, an᠆ chicken wings. But you are breaking the cycle now, and that's w᠆ ᠆ matters.

We can all look a᠆ ᠆nd and see obesity, heart disease, diabetes, cancer, osteoporosi᠆ ᠆nd other diet-related illnesses touching more lives than ever ᠆ ᠆re. By switching to a plant-based diet you'll be taking or ᠆omentous leap toward avoiding these serious conditions

In wc ᠆ng with research participants, dietitians at the Physicians C ᠆mittee for Responsible Medicine have found the greatest succe᠆ with women who follow this eating plan 100 percent. An eas᠆ ᠆ay to ensure that you will stick with it is to commit yourself c ᠆pletely for three weeks. There's no need to follow the daily ᠆nus exactly; just choose any of the recipes that appeal to you. At ᠆e end of this time, many people are anxious to explore more new ᠆astes and are already enjoying the benefits of a vegan diet. Three weeks will easily turn to months, and then to years.

Speaking of years, the clock is ticking for all of us. Yet when you change your eating habits in as dramatic a way as this, you'll begin to see each day as an opportunity for strengthening and invigorating your cells, your body, *your life*. Father Time will surely smile upon you. So get going and enjoy!

We wish you the very best of success in your new endeavor, and the very best of health.

14

Cooking Tips
and Techniques

Whether you're cooking for a family, for two, or just for yourself, the following recipes and menus will help you prepare delicious, healthful meals that will please everyone. You'll find practical suggestions for menu planning and shopping, and sample menus based on the recipes in this book. "Stocking Your Pantry" provides suggestions for staple ingredients as well as convenient instant meals to keep on hand, and the Glossary lists foods that may be new to you. The recipes included in this chapter are quick and easy to prepare, with ingredients that are available in most grocery stores. Many of the recipes are for healthful versions of familiar foods, and each of the recipes includes a nutrient analysis.

Planning a Menu

Planning ahead is the key to easy meal preparation. You will be amazed at the amount of time and money you save when you plan weekly menus and shop for a week at a time. You'll spend less time looking for parking and standing in line, and by planning ahead you'll spend less money on impulse items and instant meals. You'll also be delighted when you begin cooking that all the ingredients you need will be on hand.

Set aside a bit of time and find a quiet spot to plan a one-week menu. Your menu plan does not have to specify every item for every meal. Breakfasts, especially during the week, probably will be much the same from day to day: fruits, whole grain cereals, and breads. For lunches, leftovers make perfect instant meals. Soup (either homemade or commercially prepared) is another quick and nutritious option. Add whole grain bread and salad mix sprinkled with seasoned rice vinegar for a meal in minutes! Bean or grain salads are also excellent lunch foods that can be prepared in quantity and kept on hand for a quick meal. Thus your lunch menu plan should include a couple of soups and two or three salads. For dinners, plan four main dishes prepared in large enough quantities to provide at least two meals. Add whole grains such as brown rice or bulgur wheat, and vegetables for complete, satisfying meals.

A Sample Menu Plan

This flexible menu plan does not specify exact meals for each day of the week. The indicated meals can be prepared according to your time and taste. At the same time, it provides you with the assurance that the ingredients for any of the meals will be available when you need them. Use this menu plan to make a shopping list.

SAMPLE MENU PLAN

Breakfasts
   fresh fruit: blueberries, cantaloupe, oranges
   toast: whole wheat raisin, multigrain
   hot cereal: oatmeal, 10-grain cereal, cracked wheat
   cold cereal: shredded wheat, Tropical Granola
   Buckwheat Corn cakes

Lunches

soups: Black Bean Soup, African Bean Soup, Portuguese Kale
   Soup

salads: Four Bean Salad, Spinach Salad with Curry Dressing,
   Tabouli

Dinners

Hearty Barbecue Beans
Polenta
Green salad with Piquant Dressing

Red Lentil Curry
Brown Rice
Broccoli with Sun-Dried Tomatoes

Pan-Seared Portobello Mushrooms
Polenta
Braised Collards or Kale

Stuffed Eggplant
Black Bean Soup
Bulgur

Making a Shopping List

Use your menu plan to prepare a shopping list. Look up the recipes
you have chosen and note the ingredients you'll need to purchase.
Add a variety of fresh vegetables and fruits, whole grains, and
breads to round out your meals. Check the refrigerator, freezer, and
pantry to see what staples need to be restocked (see "Stocking Your
Pantry" on page 158). These might include condiments, spices,
baking supplies, canned foods, frozen foods, or beverages.

To streamline your shopping trip, arrange the foods on your list
in categories that reflect the departments in your grocery store, such
as fresh produce, grains, dried beans, canned fruits and vegetables,
and frozen foods.

SAMPLE SHOPPING LIST

Fresh Produce

oranges	portobello	collard greens
bananas	mushrooms	zucchini
cantaloupes	sweet potatoes	avocados
blueberries	green onions	yellow onions
other seasonal	green beans	red onions
fruits	green bell peppers	garlic
prewashed salad	red bell peppers	jicamas
mix	tomatoes	other seasonal
prewashed spinach	fresh beets	vegetables
carrots	red potatoes	
celery	broccoli	

Breakfast Cereals

oatmeal	multigrain cereals	shredded wheat

Grains and Pasta

rolled oats	polenta	buckwheat flour
couscous	whole wheat pastry	cornmeal
brown basmati rice	flour	elbow macaroni

Dried Beans, and Peas

lentils	pinto beans	split peas

Canned Vegetables and Fruits

15-ounce can diced beets	15-ounce can kidney beans	roasted red peppers
28-ounce can crushed tomatoes	15-ounce can garbanzo beans	tomato juice

Packaged Foods

ramen soups	fortified soy milk or rice milk	maple syrup

Refrigerated Foods

tofu	flour tortillas

Bread
   whole wheat bread

Salad Dressing, Vinegar, and Condiments
   soy sauce   balsamic vinegar

Herbs and Spices
   chili powder   oregano

Frozen Foods
   orange juice   apple juice   chopped spinach
   concentrate   concentrate

Seasonal Eating

Seasonal eating refers to choosing fruits and vegetables when they are fresh and in season. By doing so, you will enjoy better-tasting, more nutritious produce and cut your food costs at the same time. Seasonal produce tastes better because it is usually picked at its prime. It hasn't spent weeks in transit from the other side of the equator, or months in cold storage where it loses moisture, flavor, and nutrients. Ironically, transportation and cold storage, which detract from the flavor and nutritional value of produce, add significantly to its cost.

There are a number of ways to know what foods are in season. Seasonal foods are usually featured in advertisements and in the produce department at your market. Check your store's advertising flyer and look for large end-aisle displays in the produce department. In general you will find that seasonal foods are more reasonably priced than out-of-season produce because of lower storage, shipping, and handling costs. You will also find that when foods are in season, there are often several varieties to choose from. For example, when apples get ripe in autumn, most stores feature several varieties. By spring and summer, however, only the few varieties that can be held in cold storage are available.

Farmers' markets offer an enjoyable way to find out what is in season. The produce at farmers' markets is not only seasonal, but is often organically grown as well. An easy way to obtain seasonal produce is to join a CSA (community-supported agriculture), in which you pay a fee to a local grower who then supplies you with a variety of fresh produce throughout the season. At www.umass.edu/umext/csa/us/StateList.html you can get more information about CSAs, including local listings.

The most basic way of knowing what is in season is to consider what part of the plant a food comes from. During the colder months, foods that are in season generally come from the roots, stems, and leaves of plants. As the weather warms, pods, flowers, and eventually fruits come into season. Fruit, by the way, refers to the seed-bearing portion of a plant and includes such foods as tomatoes, peppers, avocados, squash, and eggplant.

Stocking Up

With your shopping list in hand, you will be ready to stock up quickly and conveniently for the whole week. Make sure you have eaten before you head for the store. Shopping on an empty stomach can override the best of intentions and lead to impulsive purchases of less-than-nutritious foods.

Most processed foods have nutrition labels and ingredient lists that provide you with useful information for making healthy food choices. The nutrition label indicates the size of a single serving and the number of calories as well as the amount of fat, protein, sugar, fiber, and salt in that serving. You can also gather a lot of useful information by reading through the ingredients list. The ingredients are listed in order of prominence in the food: the ingredient present in the greatest amount is first on the list, and so forth. Thus, if fat or sugar appears near the top of the list, you know that these are major ingredients. The ingredients list also indicates the presence of artificial flavors, artificial colors, preservatives, and other additives you may wish to avoid.

As you read through the ingredients list, be aware of the many different forms of sugar that may be in food. Sucrose, fructose, dextrose, corn syrup, honey, and malt are just a few, and in general, any ingredients that end with "-ose" are sugars. If a product contains several different types of sugar it is likely that sugar is a major ingredient, even if it isn't the first item on the list.

You should also avoid foods that contain hydrogenated oils. These oils have been processed to make them solid, or saturated, and like other saturated fats, they can raise blood cholesterol levels and increase the risk of heart disease.

In addition to nutrition labels and ingredients lists, foods may contain other nutrition claims, such as "fat-free," "low cholesterol," or "lite." The definition of these terms, as outlined by the U.S. Food and Drug Administration, are given in the following list.

Light (lite). May refer to calories, fat, or sodium. Contains a third fewer calories, or no more than half the fat of the higher-calorie, higher-fat version; or no more than half the sodium of the higher-sodium version.

Calorie-free. Contains fewer than 5 calories per serving.

Fat-free. Contains fewer than 0.5 gram of fat per serving.

Low-fat. Contains 3 grams (or less) of fat per serving.

Reduced or less fat. At least 25 percent less fat per serving than the higher-fat version.

Cholesterol-free. Contains fewer than 2 milligrams of cholesterol and 2 grams (or less) of saturated fat per serving.

Low cholesterol. Contains 20 milligrams (or less) of cholesterol and 2 grams (or less) of saturated fat per serving.

Reduced cholesterol. At least 25 percent less cholesterol than the higher-cholesterol version and 2 grams (or less) or saturated fat per serving.

Sodium-free. Contains fewer than 5 milligrams of sodium per serving and no sodium chloride in ingredients.

Very low sodium. Contains 35 milligrams (or less) of sodium per serving.

Low sodium. Contains 140 milligrams (or less) of sodium per serving.

Stocking Your Pantry

BASIC INGREDIENTS AND QUICK FOODS

Produce

yellow onions
red onions
garlic
red potatoes
russet potatoes
green cabbage

carrots, baby carrots
celery
prewashed salad mix
prewashed spinach

broccoli
kale or collard greens
apples
oranges
bananas

Grains and Grain Products

short grain brown rice
long grain brown rice
bulgur
whole wheat flour
whole wheat pastry flour

unbleached flour
potato flour
rice flour
barley flour
whole wheat couscous
rolled oats
polenta

cornmeal
eggless pasta
cold breakfast cereals without added fat or sugars
hot breakfast cereals

Dried Beans, Lentils, and Peas

pinto beans
black beans
lentils

split peas
black bean flakes: Fantastic Foods, Taste Adventure

pinto bean flakes: Fantastic Foods, Taste Adventure

Canned Foods

basic beans (pinto, garbanzo, kidney, black)
prepared beans (vegetarian chili, baked beans, refried beans)

tomato products (crushed tomatoes, tomato sauce, tomato paste)
vegetables (corn, beets, water-packed roasted red peppers)

vegetarian soups
vegetarian pasta sauce (preferably fat-free)
salsa

Frozen Foods

unsweetened juice concentrates (apple, orange, white grape) frozen bananas	frozen berries frozen vegetables (corn, peas, Italian green beans, broccoli)	chopped onions frozen diced bell peppers

Nuts, Seeds, and Dried Fruit

peanut butter	tahini (sesame butter)	raisins

Breads, Crackers, and Snack Foods

whole grain bread (may be frozen) whole wheat pita bread	corn tortillas (may be frozen) whole wheat tortillas (may be frozen)	fat-free snack foods (crackers, rice cakes, popcorn cakes, baked tortilla chips, pretzels)

Convenience Foods

vegetarian soup cups vegetarian ramen soups	silken tofu vegetarian burgers, cold cuts, hot dogs	baked tofu textured vegetable protein

Condiments and Seasonings

herbs and spices reduced-sodium soy sauce cider vinegar balsamic vinegar seasoned rice vinegar vegetable broth vegetable oil spray	molasses maple syrup raw or turbinado sugar baking soda low-sodium baking powder (Featherweight) spreadable fruit	fat-free salad dressing eggless mayonnaise (Vegenaise, Nayonaise) stone-ground mustard catsup

Beverages

fortified soy milk or rice milk	hot beverages (herbal teas, Cafix, Postum, Pero)

Meal Preparation

With your menu and ingredients on hand, you will be able to prepare satisfying meals quickly and conveniently. You may wish to prepare several different menu items in a single cooking session as a further time-saver.

You will notice that most of the recipes in this book provide six to eight servings. As a result, you will probably have food left over that can be used to provide one or more extra meals. In this way the menu you create may actually provide meals for more than a week, with no additional shopping, planning, or cooking!

Another time-saver is to make slight modifications to the food you've already prepared so it has a different appearance the second or third time you serve it. In this way you can have maximum variety with a minimum of preparation. The Polenta recipe (see page 178) is a good example. Start out by preparing a triple batch and have it as a creamy porridge for breakfast topped with fresh fruit and soy milk as indicated in the recipe. For a second meal, allow to cool in a flat pan overnight, and slice to make Grilled Polenta (see page 181) the next day. Then for a quick and delicious lunch use the remaining polenta to make Polenta Pizza (see page 212).

Foods that take a bit of time to cook can be prepared in large enough quantities to provide for several meals. Brown rice is a good example. Once cooked, it can easily be reheated in a microwave or on the stovetop and served as a side dish with a variety of recipes. It also can be added to soups and stews, or used as a filling in a burrito or a wrap.

Cooking Techniques

Vegetables

The secret to preparing vegetables is to cook them only as much as is needed to tenderize them and bring out their best flavor. The following methods are quick and easy and enhance the flavor and texture of vegetables.

Steaming. A collapsible steamer rack can turn any pot into a vegetable steamer. Heat about 1 inch of water in a pot. Arrange the prepared vegetables in a single layer on a steamer rack and place them in the pot over the boiling water. Cover the pot with a lid and cook until just tender.

Braising. This technique is identical to sautéing, except that a fat-free liquid is used in place of oil. It is particularly useful for mellowing the flavor of vegetables such as onions and garlic. Heat approximately ½ cup of water, vegetable broth, or wine (the liquid you use will depend on the recipe) in a large pan or skillet. Add the vegetables and cook over high heat, stirring occasionally, adding small amounts of additional liquid if needed, until the vegetables are tender. This will take about five minutes for onions.

Grilling. High heat seals in the flavors of vegetables and adds its own distinctive flavor as well. Vegetables can be grilled on a barbecue or electric grill, or on the stove using a nonstick grill pan. Cut all the foods that will be grilled together into a uniform size. Preheat the grill, then add the vegetables. Cook over medium-high heat, turning occasionally with a spatula until uniformly browned and tender.

Roasting. A simple and delicious way to prepare vegetables is to roast them in a very hot oven (450°F). Toss the vegetables with seasonings and a small amount of olive oil if desired. Spread them in a single layer on a baking sheet and place them in the preheated oven until tender.

Microwave. A microwave oven provides an easy method for cooking vegetables, particularly those that take a long time to cook with other methods. Another benefit of microwave cooking for vegetables is that they cook quickly with little or no water, minimizing loss of nutrients. Try the recipes for yams, potatoes, and winter squash on page 224.

Grains

Whole grains are a mainstay of a healthful diet. The term "whole grain" refers to grains that have been minimally processed, leaving the bran and germ intact. As a result, whole grains provide significantly more nutrients, including protein, vitamins, and minerals, than refined grains. In addition, whole grains are an excellent source of fiber. Some fairly common whole grains include whole wheat berries, cracked wheat and bulgur, whole wheat flour, brown rice, rolled oats, whole barley, and barley flour. Some of the less common grains that are slowly making their way into the mainstream are quinoa ("keen-wah"), amaranth, kamut ("kam-oo"), and teff.

Grains should be stored in a cool, dry location. If the outer bran layer has been disturbed by crushing or grinding, as in making flour or rolled oats, the grain should be used within two to three months. Grains with the outer bran layer intact remain viable and nutritious for several years if properly stored.

When cooking grains, the following tips are useful:

- The easiest way to cook most grains is to simmer them, loosely covered, on the stovetop.
- Lightly roasting grains in a dry skillet before cooking enhances their nutty flavor and gives them a lighter texture. The flavor of millet is particularly enhanced by roasting.
- Grains should not be stirred during cooking, unless the recipe indicates otherwise. They will be lighter and fluffier if left alone.
- When cooking grains, make enough for several meals. Cooked grains can be reheated in a microwave or on the stovetop.
- An easy way to reheat grains on the stove is to place them in a vegetable steamer over boiling water.
- Fine-textured grains such as couscous and bulgur are actually fluffier when they are not cooked. Simply pour boiling water over the grain, then cover and let stand for fifteen to twenty minutes. Fluff the grain with a fork before serving.

Legumes

The term "legume" refers to dried beans and peas such as soybeans, black beans, pinto beans, garbanzos or chickpeas, lentils, and split peas. Legumes may be purchased dried, canned, and in some cases, frozen or dehydrated. Dried beans are inexpensive and easy to cook. If you don't have the time to cook dried beans, canned beans are a good alternative. Kidney beans, garbanzo beans, pinto beans, black beans, and many others are available, including some in low-sodium varieties. For an even quicker meal, vegetarian baked beans, chili beans, and refried beans are available in the canned foods section of most supermarkets.

Recently a few companies have introduced precooked, dehy-drated beans. These cook in about five minutes. Pinto beans, black beans, split peas, and lentils are some of the varieties available. Check your local natural food store for these.

Note the following tips for cooking dried beans:

- Sort through the beans, discard any debris, then rinse thoroughly.
- Soaking beans before cooking reduces their cooking time and increases their digestibility. Soak at least four hours, then pour off soak water and add fresh water for cooking.
- Cook in a large pot with plenty of water. Cover the pot loosely. Use medium-low heat to maintain a low simmer. Check occasionally, adding more water if needed.
- A Crock-Pot is an ideal place to cook beans. The slow, even heat ensures thorough cooking. Start with boiling water and use the highest setting for quickest cooking. For slower cooking, start with cold water and use the highest setting.
- Beans can be cooked very quickly in a pressure cooker. Follow the instructions that came with the cooker.
- Beans should be thoroughly cooked. They should smash easily when pressed between thumb and forefinger.
- Salt toughens the skins of beans and increases the cooking time. It should not be added until the beans are tender.
- Cooked beans may be frozen in airtight containers for later use.

Cutting Fat

Foods that are high in fat are also high in calories. In addition to causing unwanted weight gain, a high-fat diet increases your risk for heart disease, adult-onset diabetes, and several forms of cancer. By switching to a plant-based diet you will reduce your intake of fat considerably. The following tips will help you reduce your fat intake even further.

- Choose cooking techniques that do not employ added fat. Baking, grilling, and oven roasting are great alternatives to frying.

COOKING DRIED BEANS AND PEAS

BEANS (1 CUP DRY)	AMOUNT OF WATER	COOKING TIME	YIELD
Adzuki beans	3 cups	1½ hours	2¼ cups
Black beans	3 cups	1½ hours	2¼ cups
Black-eyed peas	3 cups	1 hour	2 cups
Chickpeas (garbanzos)	4 cups	2–3 hours	2½ cups
Great Northern beans	3½ cups	2 hours	2 cups
Kidney beans	3 cups	2 hours	2 cups
Lentils	3 cups	1 hour	2¼ cups
Lima beans	2 cups	1½ hours	1½ cups
Navy beans	3 cups	2 hours	2 cups
Pinto beans	3 cups	2½ hours	2¼ cups
Red beans	3 cups	3 hours	2 cups
Soybeans	4 cups	3 hours	2½ cups
Split peas	3 cups	1 hour	2½ cups

- Another fat-cutting cooking trick is to sauté in a liquid such as water or vegetable broth whenever possible. Heat about ½ cup of water in a skillet (preferably nonstick) and add the vegetables to be sautéed. Cook over high heat, stirring frequently, until the vegetables are tender. This will take about five minutes. Add a bit more water if necessary to prevent sticking.
- Add onions and garlic to soups and stews at the beginning of the cooking time so their flavors will mellow without sautéing.
- When oil is absolutely necessary to prevent sticking, lightly apply a vegetable oil spray. Another alternative is to start with a very small amount of oil (1 to 2 teaspoons), then add water or vegetable broth as needed to keep the food from sticking.

- Nonstick pots and pans allow foods to be prepared with little or no fat.
- Choose fat-free dressings for salads. In addition to commercially prepared dressings, seasoned rice vinegar makes a tasty fat-free dressing straight out of the bottle.
- Avoid deep-fried foods and fat-laden pastries. Check your market for low-fat and no-fat alternatives.
- Replace the oil in salad dressing recipes with seasoned rice vinegar, vegetable broth, bean cooking liquid, or water. For a thicker dressing, whisk in a small amount of potato flour.
- Sesame Seasoning (see page 200) is low in fat and delicious on grains, potatoes, and steamed vegetables. Fat-free salad dressing also may be used as a topping for cooked vegetables.
- Applesauce, mashed banana, prune purée, or canned pumpkin may be substituted for all or part of the fat in many baked goods.

Quick Meal and Snack Ideas

- Fresh soybeans (edamame) make a delicious snack or meal addition. Find them in the frozen vegetables section of your supermarket and prepare according to package directions.
- For an instant green salad use prewashed salad mix and commercially prepared fat-free dressing. Add some canned kidney beans or garbanzo beans for a more substantial meal.
- Baby carrots make a convenient, healthful snack. Try them plain or with Red Pepper Hummus (see page 195).
- Ramen soup is quick and satisfying. Add some chopped, fresh vegetables for a heartier soup.
- Keep a selection of vegetarian soup cups on hand. These are great for quick meals, especially when you're traveling.
- Burritos are quick to make and very portable. They can be eaten hot or cold. For a simple burrito, spread fat-free refried beans on a flour tortilla, add prewashed salad mix and salsa, and roll it up.
- Mix fat-free refried beans with an equal amount of salsa for a delicious bean dip. Serve with baked tortilla chips or fresh vegetables.

- Tofu Tacos (see page 186) are quick and easy to make. Serve them with Four Bean Salad (see page 192).

- A wide variety of fat-free vegetarian cold cuts are available in many supermarkets and natural food stores. These make quick and easy sandwiches.

- Rice cakes and popcorn cakes make great snack foods. Spread them with Red Pepper Hummus (see page 195), apple butter, or spreadable fruit.

- Drain garbanzo beans and spoon onto a piece of pita bread. Top with prewashed salad mix and fat-free salad dressing for a quick pocket sandwich.

- Heat a fat-free vegetarian burger patty in the toaster oven. Serve it on a whole grain bun with mustard, ketchup or barbecue sauce, and lettuce. Add sliced red onion and tomato if desired.

- Keep baked or steamed potatoes in the refrigerator. For a quick meal, heat a potato in the microwave and top it with salsa or Broccoli with Sun-Dried Tomatoes (see page 221) or Black Bean Hash (see page 211).

- Arrange chunks of fresh fruit on skewers for quick fruit kabobs.

- Frozen grapes make a refreshing summer snack. To prepare, remove them from the stems and freeze, loosely packed, in an airtight container.

- Frozen bananas make cool snacks or creamy desserts. Peel the bananas, break into chunks, and freeze in airtight containers.

15

Menus for a Week

DAY 1

Breakfast

    Tropical Granola (page 171)

    fortified soy milk or rice milk

    fresh fruit

    herb tea

Lunch

    Tofu, Lettuce, and Tomato Sandwich (page 183)

    Four Bean Salad (page 192)

    fresh fruit

Dinner

    Red Lentil Curry (page 208)

    Brown Rice (page 176)

    Green salad with Piquant Dressing (page 196)

    Cranberry Apple Crisp (page 230)

DAY 2

Breakfast

 Cinnamon Raisin French Toast (page 175)
 Corn Butter (page 201)
 maple syrup or spreadable fruit
 fresh fruit
 herb tea

Lunch

 African Bean Soup (page 203)
 Spinach Salad with Curry Dressing (page 194)
 whole grain bread

Dinner

 Stuffed Eggplant (page 218)
 Black Bean Soup (page 206)
 Garlic Bread (page 226)
 Fruit Gel (page 233)

DAY 3

Breakfast

 Multigrain Cereal (page 172)
 fortified soy milk or rice milk
 fresh fruit
 herb tea

Lunch

 Three Sisters Salad (page 190)
 corn tortillas
 watermelon

Dinner

 Instant Falafel Pockets (page 188) with Cool Cucumber Sauce
   (page 199)
 Tabouli (page 195)
 Braised Collards or Kale (page 219)
 Pumpkin Raisin Cookies (231)

Day 4

Breakfast

Buckwheat Corncakes (page 174)
Corn Butter (page 201)
maple syrup, fresh fruit, or spreadable fruit
herb tea

Lunch

Portuguese Kale Soup (page 203)
whole grain bread or roll
Brown Rice Salad (page 192)

Dinner

Mexican Skillet Pie (page 208)
green salad
Peach Smoothie (page 234)

Day 5

Breakfast

Breakfast Scramble (page 174)
whole grain toast
fresh fruit
herb tea

Lunch

Chili Potato Soup (page 204)
whole grain bread or roll
Antipasto Salad (page 190)

Dinner

Tofu Brochettes (page 215)
Cucumber Salad (page 191)
Grilled Polenta (page 181)
Fat-Free Banana Cake (page 230)

DAY 6

Breakfast

Fresh Apple Muffins (page 227)

fresh fruit

herb tea

Lunch

Nori Rolls (page 188)

Broccoli and Bok Choy with Baked Tofu (page 210)

fresh fruit

Dinner

Macaroni with Creamy Tofu Sauce (page 216)

Broccoli with Sun-Dried Tomatoes (page 221)

green salad with fat-free dressing

Butterscotch Pudding (page 229)

DAY 7

Breakfast

Muesli (page 172) or other cold cereal

fortified soy milk or rice milk

fresh fruit

herb tea

Lunch

Tempeh Salad Sandwich (page 183)

baby carrots with Red Pepper Hummus (page 195)

baked tofu

Dinner

Shepherd's Pie (page 213)

Bok Choy (page 220)

green salad with Balsamic Vinaigrette (page 196)

Tofu Cheesecake (page 232)

16

The Recipes

BREAKFASTS

Tropical Granola

MAKES ABOUT 5 CUPS (10 ½-CUP SERVINGS)

This granola is sweetened with dried fruit and maple syrup.

3 cups rolled oats or other rolled grains	¼ cup diced dried papaya
⅓ cup sunflower seeds	¼ cup diced dried pineapple
⅓ cup sliced almonds	¼ cup golden or sultana raisins
⅓ cup cashews	½ cup maple syrup
	1 teaspoon coconut extract

Preheat oven to 350°F.

Mix rolled oats, sunflower seeds, almonds, cashews, papaya, pineapple, and raisins in a large bowl. Add maple syrup and coconut extract. Mix completely.

Spread in thin layers on two large baking sheets and bake until edges begin to turn golden. Use a spatula to turn and continue baking until granola is dry and crispy, about 20 minutes altogether.

Remove from oven and cool. Transfer to an airtight container for storage.

Per ½-cup serving: 233 calories; 7 g protein; 37 g carbohydrate; 8 g fat;
4 g fiber; 5 mg sodium; calories from protein: 11%;
calories from carbohydrates: 61%; calories from fats: 28%

* * *

Muesli

MAKES ABOUT 3 CUPS OF MUESLI (6 ½-CUP SERVINGS)

Muesli, a European breakfast standard, is made from uncooked grains traditionally soaked in fruit juice overnight. Try this updated morning treat with rolled oats that can be eaten right away.

2 cups rolled oats	½ cup chopped dried fruit (apples,
¼ cup chopped almonds	figs, apricots, etc.)
	½ cup raisins

Combine oats, almonds, dried fruit, and raisins. Leave whole or grind in a food processor for a finer cereal.

To serve, mix with hot or cold fortified soy milk or rice milk, fruit juice, or applesauce. Top with fresh fruit if desired, and let stand a few minutes before serving.

Store in an airtight container in the refrigerator.

Per ½-cup serving: 202 calories; 6 g protein; 36 g carbohydrate;
5 g fat; 4 g fiber; 5 mg sodium; calories from protein: 12%;
calories from carbohydrates: 68%; calories from fats: 20%

* * *

Multigrain Cereal

MAKES 2½ 1-CUP SERVINGS

Multigrain hot cereals provide great flavor as well as the nutritional benefits of several whole grains. A variety of multigrain cereal mixes are available in natural food stores and many supermarkets. One of the most delicious and most widely distributed is Bob's Red Mill 10 Grain Cereal (see Glossary). Use this method for cooking any of these hearty, satisfying breakfast cereals.

1 cup multigrain cereal mix	3 cups boiling water
½ teaspoon salt (optional)	

Stir cereal and salt into boiling water in a saucepan. Cover loosely and simmer, stirring occasionally, for 7 minutes.

Remove from heat and let stand, covered, for 10 minutes before serving.

Health hint: By gradually reducing the amount of salt you add, you can reeducate your taste buds so that the cereal will taste fine with no salt at all.

Per 1-cup serving: 200 calories; 6 g protein; 40 g carbohydrate;
2 g fat; 4 g fiber; 10 to 580 mg sodium (depending on amount
of salt used in recipe); calories from protein: 13%;
calories from carbohydrates: 77%; calories from fats: 10%

● ● ●

Rolled Grain Cereal
MAKES 2 1-CUP SERVINGS

Everyone is familiar with rolled oats, but several other whole grains are available in this easy-to-cook form. Check your natural food store or supermarket for rolled wheat, rye, barley, or triticale. Some are sold in boxes in the cereal section, and others may be found in the bulk food department. These can be cooked individually or mixed to make a multigrain cereal.

2   cups boiling water $\frac{1}{4}$ teaspoon salt (optional)
1   cup rolled grain cereal

Add cereal and salt to boiling water in a saucepan. Reduce heat to a simmer, cover loosely, and cook 7 minutes.

Remove from heat and let stand, covered, for 5 minutes before serving.

Per 1-cup serving (of rolled wheat): 146 calories;
4 g protein; 32 g carbohydrate; 0.8 g fat; 4 g fiber;
0–268 mg sodium; ; calories from protein: 12%;
calories from carbohydrates: 83%; calories from fats: 5%

● ● ●

Blueberry Barley Breakfast
MAKES 2 1-CUP SERVINGS

This is a delicious way to enjoy leftover Brown Rice and Barley (page 177).

1   cup Brown Rice and Barley, hot   1   cup fortified vanilla soy milk or
    or cold   rice milk
1   cup blueberries, fresh or frozen   3   tablespoons maple syrup

Heat Brown Rice and Barley if desired, then add blueberries, milk, and maple syrup. Stir to mix.

Per 1-cup serving: 324 calories; 8 g protein; 70 g carbohydrate;
2 g fat; 9 g fiber; 174 mg sodium; calories from protein: 9%;
calories from carbohydrates: 84%; calories from fats: 7%

● ● ●

Breakfast Scramble

MAKES 4 1-CUP SERVINGS

Enjoy the benefits of soy with this tofu breakfast. Delicious with toast and Apple Chutney (page 198).

2 teaspoons olive oil or toasted sesame oil
1 small onion, chopped
2 cups sliced mushrooms

1 pound firm tofu, cut into ½-inch dice
1½ teaspoons curry powder
2 tablespoons reduced-sodium soy sauce

Heat oil in a large nonstick skillet, then sauté onion and mushrooms over high heat, stirring often, until onion is soft, about 5 minutes.

Add tofu, curry powder, and soy sauce. Continue cooking another 5 minutes.

Variation: For a more elaborate scramble, add additional chopped vegetables such as carrots, celery, peppers, or green onions.

Per 1-cup serving: 127 calories; 11 g protein; 6 g carbohydrate;
8 g fat; 2 g fiber; 524 mg sodium; calories from protein: 31%;
calories from carbohydrates: 18%; calories from fats: 51%

• • •

Buckwheat Corncakes

MAKES 16 3-INCH PANCAKES

Buckwheat adds a wonderful, hearty flavor to these easily prepared pancakes. Serve them with homemade applesauce, fresh fruit, or maple syrup.

½ cup buckwheat flour
½ cup cornmeal
½ teaspoon sodium-free baking powder
¼ teaspoon baking soda
¼ teaspoon salt
1 ripe banana, mashed

2 tablespoons maple syrup
1 tablespoon white or cider vinegar
1 cup fortified soy milk or rice milk
vegetable oil cooking spray

Mix buckwheat flour, cornmeal, baking powder, baking soda, and salt.

In a large bowl, combine mashed banana, maple syrup, vinegar, and milk. Add flour mixture, stirring just enough to remove any lumps and make a pourable batter. Add a bit more milk if batter seems too thick.

Preheat a nonstick skillet or griddle, then spray lightly with vegetable oil. Pour a scant ¼ cup of batter onto the heated surface and cook until tops bubble. Turn carefully with a spatula and cook the second sides until browned, about 1 minute. Serve immediately.

Per corncake: 44 calories; 1 g protein; 9 g carbohydrate;
0.5 g fat; 1 g fiber; 56 mg sodium; calories from protein: 11%;
calories from carbohydrates: 79%; calories from fats: 10%

● ● ●

Oatmeal Waffles

MAKES 6 WAFFLES

*These easily prepared waffles are a delicious way to add healthful oats to
your diet.*

2 cups rolled oats	1 teaspoon vanilla
2 cups water	fresh fruit, spreadable fruit or
1 banana	maple syrup for serving
¼ teaspoon salt	vegetable oil cooking spray
1 tablespoon maple syrup	

Preheat waffle iron to medium-high.

Combine oats, water, banana, salt, maple syrup, and vanilla in a
blender. Blend on high speed until completely smooth.

Lightly spray waffle iron with cooking spray. Pour in enough batter to
just barely reach edges and cook until golden brown, 5 to 10 minutes,
without lifting lid.

Note: The batter should be pourable. If it becomes too thick as it
stands, add a bit more water to achieve desired consistency.

Serve with fresh fruit, spreadable fruit, or syrup.

Per waffle: 130 calories; 5 g protein; 25 g carbohydrate; 2 g fat; 3 g fiber;
90 mg sodium; calories from protein: 14%;
calories from carbohydrates: 74%; calories from fats: 12%

● ● ●

Cinnamon Raisin French Toast

MAKES 6 SLICES

*This cholesterol-free French toast is a delicious way to start the day, and
it adds beneficial soy and whole wheat to your diet.*

1 cup fortified soy milk or rice	1 teaspoon vanilla
milk (plain or vanilla)	½ teaspoon cinnamon
¼ cup whole wheat pastry flour	6 slices cinnamon raisin bread
1 tablespoon maple syrup	vegetable oil cooking spray

Combine milk, flour, maple syrup, vanilla, and cinnamon in a blender.
Blend until smooth, then pour into a flat dish.

Soak bread slices in batter until soft but not soggy. The amount of
time this takes will vary depending on the bread used.

Cook in an oil-sprayed nonstick skillet until first side is golden brown, about 3 minutes. Turn carefully with a spatula and cook second side until brown, about 3 minutes.

Per slice: 129 calories; 6 g protein; 23 g carbohydrate;
2 g fat; 4 g fiber; 191 mg sodium; calories from protein: 17%;
calories from carbohydrates: 68%; calories from fats: 15%

● ● ●

Banana Oat French Toast
MAKES 6 SLICES

Serve this delicious, heart-healthy French toast with maple syrup and fresh fruit.

1 cup fortified vanilla soy milk
¼ cup quick-cooking rolled oats
1 medium banana

6 slices whole grain bread
vegetable oil cooking spray

Combine soy milk, rolled oats, and banana in a blender. Process until completely smooth, 2 to 3 minutes. Transfer to a shallow dish.

Soak bread slices in batter until soft but not soggy. The amount of time this takes will vary depending on the bread used.

Cook over medium-high heat in an oil-sprayed nonstick skillet until first side is golden brown, about 3 minutes. Turn carefully with a spatula and cook second side until brown, about 3 minutes.

Per slice: 126 calories; 5 g protein; 24 g carbohydrate;
2 g fat; 3 g fiber; 184 mg sodium; calories from protein: 14%;
calories from carbohydrates: 73%; calories from fats: 13%

GRAINS AND PASTA
Brown Rice
MAKES 3 1-CUP SERVINGS OF COOKED RICE

Flavorful and satisfying, brown rice is an excellent source of protective soluble fiber. In the cooking method described below, the rice is toasted, then simmered in plenty of water (like pasta) to enhance its flavor and reduce cooking time.

1 cup short- or long-grain brown
   rice

4 cups boiling water
½ teaspoon salt

Rinse rice in cool water. Drain off as much water as possible.

Place rice in a saucepan over medium heat, stirring constantly until completely dry, 3 to 5 minutes.

Add boiling water and salt, then cover and simmer until rice is just tender, about 35 minutes. Pour off excess liquid (this can be saved and used as a broth for soups and stews if desired).

Per 1-cup serving: 228 calories; 5 g protein; 48 g carbohydrate; 2 g fat; 2 g fiber; 360 mg sodium; calories from protein: 9%; calories from carbohydrates: 84%; calories from fats: 7%

* * *

Brown Rice and Barley
MAKES ABOUT 6 CUPS (6 1-CUP SERVINGS)

The addition of whole barley adds great texture to brown rice. Hulled barley, which is a bit less refined and slightly more nutritious than pearled barley, is sold in many natural food stores.

1   cup short-grain brown rice
1   cup hulled or pearled barley

1   teaspoon salt
4 cups boiling water

Bring 4 cups water to a boil; add rice, barley, and salt. Reduce heat to a simmer, then cover and cook until grains are tender and all the water is absorbed, about 45 minutes.

Per 1-cup serving: 222 calories; 6 g protein; 46 g carbohydrate; 2 g fat; 6 g fiber; 362 mg sodium; calories from protein: 11%; calories from carbohydrates: 81%; calories from fats: 8%

* * *

Bulgur
MAKES 2½ CUPS (2 1-CUP SERVINGS)

Bulgur is made from whole wheat kernels that have been cracked and toasted, giving it a delicious, nutty flavor. It cooks quickly and may be served plain, or in a pilaf or salad. It is sold in natural food stores, and in some supermarkets, usually in the bulk food section.

1   cup uncooked bulgur
½ teaspoon salt

2   cups boiling water

Mix bulgur and salt in a large bowl. Stir in boiling water. Cover and let stand until tender, about 25 minutes.

Alternate cooking method: Stir bulgur and salt into boiling water in a saucepan.

Reduce heat to a simmer, then cover and cook without stirring until bulgur is tender, about 15 minutes.

Per 1-cup serving: 192 calories; 6 g protein; 42 g carbohydrate;
0.8 g fat; 10 g fiber; 436 mg sodium; calories from protein: 13%;
calories from carbohydrates: 84%; calories from fats: 3%

• • •

Whole Wheat Couscous
MAKES 3 CUPS (3 1-CUP SERVINGS)

*Couscous is actually pasta that takes only minutes to prepare. It makes a
delicious side dish or salad base. Whole wheat couscous, which contains
fiber and more vitamins and minerals than refined couscous, is sold in
natural food stores and some supermarkets.*

1 cup whole wheat couscous   1½ cups boiling water
½ teaspoon salt

Stir couscous and salt into boiling water in a saucepan. Remove from heat
and cover. Let stand 10 to 15 minutes, then fluff with a fork and serve.

Per 1-cup serving: 200 calories; 6 g protein; 42 g carbohydrate;
0.2 g fat; 4 g fiber; 364 mg sodium; calories from protein: 14%;
calories from carbohydrates: 85%; calories from fats: 1%

• • •

Polenta
MAKES 4 CUPS (4 1-CUP SERVINGS)

*Polenta, or coarsely ground cornmeal, is easy to prepare and tremen-
dously versatile. When it is first cooked it is soft, like Cream of Wheat, and
perfect for breakfast topped with fruit and fortified soy milk, or for dinner
topped with vegetables and a savory sauce. When chilled, it becomes firm
and sliceable, perfect for grilling or sautéing.*

5 cups water   1 teaspoon thyme (optional)
1 cup polenta   1 teaspoon oregano (optional)
1 teaspoon salt

Measure water into a large pot, then whisk in polenta, salt, and herbs, if
using.

Simmer over medium heat, stirring often, until very thick, about
25 minutes.

Serve hot or transfer to a 9-by-13-inch baking dish and chill until firm.

For grilled polenta, turn cold polenta out of the pan onto a cutting
board and cut it with a sharp knife into ½-inch-thick slices. Lightly spray
a large nonstick skillet with vegetable oil cooking spray and place it over
medium-high heat. Arrange polenta slices in a single layer about 1 inch

apart and cook 5 minutes. Turn and cook second side 5 minutes. Repeat with remaining polenta.

Per 1-cup serving: 110 calories; 2 g protein; 23 g carbohydrate;
2 g fiber; 1 g fat; 592 mg sodium; calories from protein: 9%;
calories from carbohydrates: 82%; calories from fats: 9%

• • •

Quinoa
MAKES 3 CUPS (3 1-CUP SERVINGS)

Quinoa ("keen-wah") comes from the high plains of the Andes Mountains, where it is nicknamed "the mother grain" for its life-giving properties. The National Academy of Sciences has called quinoa "one of the best sources of protein in the vegetable kingdom," because of its excellent amino acid pattern. Quinoa cooks quickly, and as it cooks the germ unfolds like a little tail. It has a light, fluffy texture, and may be eaten plain, used as a pilaf, or as an addition to soups and stews. The dry grain is coated with a bitter-tasting substance called saponin, which repels insects and birds and protects it from ultraviolet radiation. Quinoa must be washed thoroughly before cooking to remove this bitter coating. The easiest way to wash it is to place it in a strainer and rinse it with cool water until the water runs clear.

1 cup quinoa	2 cups boiling water

Rinse quinoa thoroughly in a fine sieve, then add it to boiling water in a saucepan. Reduce to a simmer, then cover loosely and cook until quinoa is tender and fluffy, about 15 minutes.

Per 1-cup serving: 212 calories; 8 g protein; 40 g carbohydrate;
4 g fat; 4 g fiber; 12 mg sodium; calories from protein: 14%;
calories from carbohydrates: 72%; calories from fats: 14%

• • •

Curried Rice
MAKES 6 1-CUP SERVINGS

Serve this beautiful golden rice with Tofu Brochette (page 215) or with steamed vegetables. Basmati and jasmine are flavorful long-grain rices that are sold in natural food stores and some supermarkets. Regular long-grain brown rice could also be used.

1 tablespoon olive oil	⅓ cup slivered almonds
1 cup brown basmati or jasmine rice	¼ teaspoon cinnamon
	⅛ teaspoon cardamom

⅛ teaspoon ginger
½ teaspoon turmeric
½ teaspoon salt

½ cup golden raisins
2 cups boiling water
1 cup frozen peas, thawed

Heat oil in a large pot. Add rice and cook over medium heat, stirring constantly, until rice becomes opaque and somewhat chalky looking, about 2 minutes.

Add almonds, cinnamon, cardamom, ginger, turmeric, and salt. Cook 2 minutes, stirring constantly.

Stir in raisins and boiling water. Cover and simmer until rice is tender and all the water is absorbed, about 60 minutes.

Stir in peas just before serving.

Per 1-cup serving: 216 calories; 5 g protein; 38 g carbohydrate;
6 g fat; 3 g fiber; 208 mg sodium; calories from protein: 9%;
calories from carbohydrates: 68%; calories from fats: 23%

●　●　●

Spicy Bulgur Pilaf
MAKES 4 1-CUP SERVINGS

Bulgur makes a quick and delicious Mexican pilaf. Serve it with refried beans or chili and a green salad.

1 tablespoon olive oil
1 medium onion, chopped
2 garlic cloves, minced
1 cup bulgur wheat
2 teaspoons chili powder
¾ teaspoon cumin

⅛ teaspoon celery seed
½ red bell pepper, seeded and
   finely diced
½ teaspoon salt
1¾ cups boiling water or Vegetable
   Broth (page 202)

Heat oil in a large skillet or pot and cook onion for 3 minutes.

Stir in garlic, bulgur, chili powder, cumin, and celery seed. Continue cooking, stirring often, until onion is soft, about 5 minutes.

Add bell pepper, salt, and boiling water. Stir to mix, then cover and simmer until bulgur is tender and all liquid is absorbed, about 20 minutes.

Oven method: Preheat oven to 350°F. Prepare as above, except before adding boiling water, transfer bulgur mixture to an ovenproof dish. Add boiling water, cover with foil and bake until bulgur is tender and all liquid is absorbed, about 30 minutes.

Per 1-cup serving: 178 calories; 6 g protein; 33 g carbohydrate;
4 g fat; 8 g fiber; 274 mg sodium; calories from protein: 11%;
calories from carbohydrates: 70%; calories from fats: 19%

●　●　●

Grilled Polenta

MAKES ABOUT 8 SLICES

Grilled polenta is delicious with a variety of foods. Try it with your favorite marinara sauce, with cooked beans, Pan-seared Portobello Mushrooms (page 215), or Braised Collards or Kale (page 219).

½ cup polenta
2 cups water
½ teaspoon salt

½ teaspoon dried rosemary, crushed
vegetable oil cooking spray

Combine polenta, water, salt, and rosemary in a saucepan and bring to a simmer. Cook, uncovered, over medium heat, stirring often, until polenta is very thick. Spread on a baking sheet in a ¼-inch thick layer and refrigerate until completely cold, about 1 hour.

Preheat broiler. Cut chilled polenta into slices (about 2-by-3 inches) and arrange on an oil-sprayed baking sheet. Place under broiler and cook until crusty, about 10 minutes. Turn and cook other side 10 minutes.

Per slice: 32 calories; 0.7 g protein; 7 g carbohydrate;
0.1 g fat; 0.6 g fiber; 133 mg sodium; calories from protein: 9%;
calories from carbohydrates: 87%; calories from fats: 4%

• • •

Savory Bread Dressing

MAKES ABOUT 4 1-CUP SERVINGS

This savory dressing is a perfect dish to take to a traditional holiday meal. Or pair it with Broccoli and Bok Choy with Baked Tofu (page 210) for a hearty feast.

1 tablespoon olive oil
1 onion, chopped
3 cups sliced mushrooms (about ½ pound)
2 celery stalks, thinly sliced
4 cups cubed whole wheat bread
⅓ cup finely chopped parsley
½ teaspoon thyme

½ teaspoon marjoram
½ teaspoon sage
½ teaspoon salt
⅛ teaspoon black pepper
1 cup (approximately) Vegetable Broth (page 202)
vegetable oil cooking spray

Heat oil in a large pot or skillet. Add onion and cook until soft and golden, about 5 minutes.

Add mushrooms and celery. Cover and cook over medium heat, stirring occasionally, for 5 minutes.

Preheat oven to 350°F.

Stir bread into onion mixture, along with parsley, thyme, marjoram, sage, salt, and black pepper. Lower heat and continue cooking 3 minutes, stirring often.

Stir in vegetable broth, a little at a time, until dressing obtains desired moistness.

Spread in an oil-sprayed baking dish. Cover and bake 20 minutes. Remove cover and bake 10 minutes longer.

Per 1-cup serving: 190 calories; 8 g protein; 32 g carbohydrate; 6 g fat; 6 g fiber; 806 mg sodium; calories from protein: 14%; calories from carbohydrates: 60%; calories from fats: 26%

• • •

Homestyle Millet with Garbanzo Gravy

MAKES ABOUT 6 1-CUP SERVINGS MILLET

MAKES ABOUT 2 CUPS GRAVY (6 ⅓-CUP SERVINGS)

The combination of millet cooked and mashed with cauliflower is surprisingly delicious—pleasing even the pickiest of palates.

Millet:
- 2 teaspoons toasted sesame oil
- 8 large garlic cloves, minced
- 1 cup millet
- 4 cups boiling water
- ½ teaspoon salt
- 1 head cauliflower (about 4 cups chopped)

Gravy:
- 2 teaspoons toasted sesame oil
- 1 small onion, chopped
- 1 15-ounce can garbanzo beans, undrained
- 2 teaspoons soy sauce
- ¼ teaspoon poultry seasoning

Heat oil in a pot, then add garlic and cook 30 seconds.

Add millet and cook 2 minutes.

Stir in boiling water and salt. Bring to a simmer, then cover and cook 10 minutes.

Add cauliflower. Cover and cook 15 minutes, stirring occasionally. Add a bit more water if mixture begins to stick.

Heat oil in a large skillet, then add onion and ¼ cup water. Cook over high heat, stirring frequently, until dry.

Add ¼ cup water, stirring to remove any bits of onion from the pan. Cook until dry and onions are lightly browned. Repeat, then transfer to a blender.

Add garbanzo beans and their liquid, soy sauce, poultry seasoning, and ½ cup water. Blend until completely smooth.

Return to skillet and heat gently, stirring occasionally, until bubbly.

Per 1-cup millet with ⅓ cup gravy: 269 calories; 9 g protein; 47 g carbohydrate; 5 g fat; 8 g fiber; 534 mg sodium; calories from protein: 13%;
calories from carbohydrates: 69%; calories from fats: 18%

SANDWICHES AND WRAPS

Tofu, Lettuce, and Tomato Sandwich (TLT)
MAKES 6 SANDWICHES

*Tofu makes a perfect "short order" sandwich in this vegetarian version of
the classic "BLT," offering all the flavor without the fat, cholesterol, or
nitrates of bacon. Be sure to use a nonstick skillet to cook the tofu.*

1 pound very firm tofu	1 to 2 tablespoons Tofu Mayo
2 teaspoons olive oil	(page 201) or other vegan
1 tablespoon soy sauce	mayonnaise
12 slices whole wheat or rye bread	6 lettuce leaves
1 to 2 tablespoons stone-ground	6 tomato slices
mustard	

Cut tofu into six slices, each about ¼-inch thick.

Heat oil in a large nonstick skillet. Add tofu and cook over medium
heat until golden brown, about 3 minutes. Turn and cook second side until
golden brown. Turn off heat. Sprinkle tofu with soy sauce, flipping it to
coat both sides.

Toast bread and spread it lightly with mustard and Tofu Mayo. Top
with slices of tofu, lettuce, tomato, and bread. Serve immediately.

Per sandwich: 255 calories; 14 g protein; 38 g carbohydrate;
7 g fat; 6 g fiber; 439 mg sodium; calories from protein: 20%;
calories from carbohydrates: 56%; calories from fats: 24%

* * *

Tempeh Salad Sandwich
MAKES 6 SANDWICHES

*Tempeh, made from whole soybeans, is sold in natural food stores and
some supermarkets. It has a firm texture that works nicely in this
sandwich spread. For a slightly different meal, serve this sandwich filling
on a bed of lettuce, garnished with tomatoes.*

8 ounces tempeh
3 tablespoons Tofu Mayo (page
   201) or other vegan mayonnaise
2 teaspoons prepared mustard
2 green onions, chopped, including green tops

1 stalk celery, diced
1 tablespoon pickle relish
1/4 teaspoon salt
12 slices whole wheat bread
6 lettuce leaves
6 tomato slices

Steam tempeh for 20 minutes. Remove from heat. Set aside to cool.

When cool enough to handle, grate tempeh and mix with Tofu Mayo, mustard, green onions, celery, pickle relish, and salt. Spread on whole wheat bread and garnish with lettuce leaves and sliced tomatoes.

Per sandwich: 268 calories; 15 g protein; 42 g carbohydrate;
6 g fat; 5 g fiber; 562 mg sodium; calories from protein: 22%;
calories from carbohydrates: 58%; calories from fats: 20%

• • •

Vegetarian Reuben Sandwich
MAKES 4 SANDWICHES

Seitan ("say-tan"), also called "wheat meat," is a high-protein, fat-free food with a meaty texture and flavor. Look for it in the deli department or freezer case of your natural food store.

1 onion, thinly sliced
2 garlic cloves, minced
1 cup sauerkraut
1 teaspoon paprika
1/2 teaspoon caraway seeds
1/2 teaspoon thyme
1/4 teaspoon black pepper

1 8-ounce package seitan, drained
   and thinly sliced
8 slices rye bread
Tofu Mayo (page 201) or other
   vegan mayonnaise
stone-ground or Dijon mustard
2 tomatoes, sliced

Heat 1/2 cup water in a large nonstick skillet and cook onion and garlic until soft, about 5 minutes.

Stir in sauerkraut, paprika, caraway seeds, thyme, and black pepper. Cook over medium heat, stirring often, for 5 minutes.

Add seitan slices. Cover and cook until heated through, about 3 minutes.

Toast bread if desired.

Spread 4 slices of bread with Tofu Mayo and mustard. Top with sauerkraut mixture, seitan slices, tomato slices, and remaining bread.

Per sandwich: 257 calories; 23 g protein; 34 g carbohydrate;
4 g fat; 6 g fiber; 523 mg sodium; calories from protein: 35%;
calories from carbohydrates: 52%; calories from fats: 13%

• • •

Meatlike Sandwiches, Burgers, and Hot Dogs

A wide variety of meatless cold cuts, burgers, and hot dogs are sold in natural food stores and most supermarkets. A sampling of these products is shown below. Check the deli case as well as the freezer section for these products and others. Be sure to read the ingredient list to determine that there are no animal ingredients, such as eggs, egg whites, cheese, whey, or casein. Check the nutritional information as well to determine the amounts of fat and sodium.

MEATLESS COLD CUTS AND DELI SLICES

Smart Bacon (Lightlife Foods)
Foney Baloney (Lightlife Foods)
Smart Deli Turkey (Lightlife Foods)
Smart Deli Bologna (Lightlife Foods)
Smart Deli Ham (Lightlife Foods)
Soylami (Lightlife Foods)
Pepperoni (Lightlife Foods)
Lean Links Sausage (Lightlife Foods)
Veggie Bologna Slices (Yves Fine Foods)
Veggie Pizza Pepperoni Slices (Yves Fine Foods)
Veggie Ham Slices (Yves Fine Foods)
Veggie Turkey Slices (Yves Fine Foods)
Veggie Salami Slices (Yves Fine Foods)

MEATLESS BURGERS

Veggie Cuisine Burger (Yves Fine Foods)
Veggie Burger Burgers (Yves Fine Foods)
Garden Vegetable Patties (Yves Fine Foods)
Black Bean and Mushroom Burgers (Yves Fine Foods)
Veggie Chick'n Burger (Yves Fine Foods)
LightBurgers (Lightlife Foods)
Prime Burger (White Wave Inc.)
Green Giant Harvest Burger (Pillsbury Company)
Vegan Original Boca Burger (Boca Burger Company)
Superburgers (Turtle Island Foods)
Natural Touch Vegan Burger (Worthington Foods)
Garden Vegan Burger (Wholesome and Hearty Foods)
Gardenburger Hamburger Style (Wholesome and Hearty Foods)

Amy's California Veggie Burger (Amy's Kitchen)
Amy's All American Burger (Amy's Kitchen)
Soy Deli All Natural Tofu Burger (Qwong Hop & Company)

MEATLESS HOT DOGS

Veggie Dogs (Yves Fine Foods)
Jumbo Veggie Dogs (Yves Fine Foods)
Hot & Spicy Jumbo Veggie Dogs
Good Dogs (Yves Fine Foods)
Tofu Dogs (Yves Fine Foods)
Smart Dogs (Lightlife Foods)
Wild Dogs (Wildwood Natural Foods)

OTHER MEATLESS PRODUCTS

Smart Ground (Lightlife Foods)
Veggie Ground Round Original (Yves Fine Foods)
Veggie Ground Round Italian (Yves Fine Foods)
Veggie Breakfast Links (Yves Fine Foods)
Canadian Veggie Bacon (Yves Fine Foods)
Veggie Breakfast Patties (Yves Fine Foods)
Chiken Chunks (Harvest Direct)
Chiken Breasts (Harvest Direct)
Tofurky Deli Slices (Turtle Island Foods)
Tofurky Jerky (Turtle Island Foods)
Not Chicken Deli Slices (United Specialty Foods)
White Wave Sandwich Slices (White Wave Foods)

Tofu Tacos

MAKES 6 TACOS

These tacos may be made with fresh or frozen tofu. Freezing tofu gives it a chewy texture, somewhat like ground beef. To freeze tofu, place it in its package in the freezer. To thaw, place it in the refrigerator. Once thawed, remove it from the package and squeeze out the excess water.

2 teaspoons olive oil
1 small onion, chopped
½ small bell pepper, diced (optional)
½ pound firm tofu, crumbled
   (about 1 cup)

1 tablespoon chili powder
1 tablespoon nutritional yeast
   (optional)
1 teaspoon garlic powder
¼ teaspoon ground cumin

¼ teaspoon ground oregano
1 tablespoon soy sauce
¼ cup tomato sauce
6 corn tortillas
1 to 2 cups shredded lettuce

2 green onions, chopped
½ cup diced tomato
⅓ cup salsa
½ avocado, sliced (optional)

Heat oil in a nonstick skillet. Add onion and bell pepper and cook over high heat, stirring often, 2 to 3 minutes.

Add tofu, chili powder, nutritional yeast, garlic powder, cumin, oregano, and soy sauce. Reduce heat to medium and cook 3 minutes, stirring often.

Add tomato sauce and cook over low heat until mixture is fairly dry, 3 to 5 minutes.

Heat a tortilla in a heavy, ungreased skillet, turning it from side to side until soft and pliable. Place a small amount of tofu mixture in the center, then fold tortilla in half and remove from heat. Garnish with lettuce, onions, tomatoes, salsa, and avocado if desired. Repeat with remaining tortillas.

Per taco: 143 calories; 6 g protein; 16 g carbohydrate;
6 g fat; 2 g fiber; 205 mg sodium; calories from protein: 16%;
alories from carbohydrates: 45%; calories from fats: 39%

Veggie Wrap
Makes 4 wraps

Veggie Wraps make a perfectly delicious, vegetable-rich meal.

¼ cup sunflower seeds
4 whole wheat tortillas
1 to 2 cups Red Pepper Hummus
   (page 195) or commercially
   prepared hummus

1 to 2 cups mixed salad greens or
   torn leaf lettuce
1 carrot, shredded
1 cup bean sprouts

Preheat oven or toaster oven to 375°F.

Place sunflower seeds in a small ovenproof dish and roast until lightly browned and fragrant, about 10 minutes. Set aside.

Warm tortillas, one at a time, in a large, dry skillet, flipping to warm both sides until soft and pliable.

Spread each tortilla evenly with about ½ cup of hummus, leaving a margin of ½ inch uncovered around the edge.

Divide remaining ingredients evenly among tortillas.

Wrap tortillas around filling.

Per wrap: 240 calories; 10 g protein; 34 g carbohydrate;
9 g fat; 4 g fiber; 240 mg sodium; calories from protein: 16%;
calories from carbohydrates: 53%; calories from fats: 31%

● ● ●

Instant Falafel Pockets
MAKES 12 SANDWICHES

These sandwiches are like Middle Eastern tacos in which pita bread (or pocket bread) takes the place of tortillas. The pita bread is filled with spicy garbanzo patties called falafel, lettuce, cucumbers, tomatoes, onions, and Cool Cucumber Sauce. Packaged mixes for falafel patties are sold in natural food stores and many supermarkets.

1   package falafel mix
6   pieces pita bread
4   cups shredded lettuce
1   cup sliced cucumber

1   medium tomato, diced
2   green onions, sliced
Cool Cucumber Sauce (page 199)

Prepare falafel patties according to package directions.

Warm pocket bread until it is soft. This may be done by placing individual pieces in a vegetable steamer over boiling water, or by wrapping it in foil and heating it in the oven.

Cut warm pita breads in half and carefully open the pockets. Fill each pita half with two falafel patties. Garnish with lettuce, cucumber, tomato, green onions, and Cool Cucumber Sauce.

Per falafel: 146 calories; 7 g protein; 27 g carbohydrate;
2 g fat; 5 g fiber; 319 mg sodium; calories from protein:
19%; calories from carbohydrates: 70%; calories from fats: 11%

● ● ●

Nori Rolls
MAKES 6 SERVINGS

Nori Rolls can be eaten like burritos, or cut into slices and arranged on a platter for a more elegant presentation. Serve with extra pickled ginger and wasabi (very hot horseradish sauce) if desired.

1   cup short-grain brown rice
¼   teaspoon salt
¼   cups seasoned rice vinegar
½   carrot, julienned or grated
½   cup thinly sliced cucumber
1   piece baked tofu, cut in thin
    strips

½ avocado, sliced
1   green onion, sliced
⅓ cup (approximately) pickled
    ginger
3   sheets nori

Combine brown rice with salt and 3 cups water in a saucepan. Cover and simmer until rice is very soft and all water has been absorbed, about 1 hour. Remove from heat and stir in vinegar. Set aside until cool.

To assemble rolls, place a sheet of nori on a cloth napkin or bamboo sushi mat. Spread with about ¾ cup of cooled rice in a thin, even layer, leaving a 1-inch band along the top uncovered.

Arrange small amounts of carrot, cucumber, tofu, avocado, and green onion on the rice. Hold filling ingredients in place with your fingertips, and use your thumbs to lift the bottom edge of the mat, so that the edge of the nori nearest you is lifted over to meet the top edge. Moisten top edge with water and use it as a "flap" to seal the roll. Use your hands to gently shape the roll, then let it sit on its seam to seal.

Per ½ roll: 176 calories; 4 g protein; 32 g carbohydrate;
4 g fat; 2 g fiber; 504 mg sodium; calories from protein: 9%;
calories from carbohydrates: 71%; calories from fats: 20%

●　●　●

Portobello and Red Pepper Wraps
MAKES 6 WRAPS

Portobello mushrooms, which are large and "meaty," make these wraps substantial and satisfying.

3 large, firm portobello mushrooms	2 garlic cloves, minced
2 teaspoons toasted sesame oil	1 cup roasted red peppers, cut into strips
2 tablespoons red wine or Vegetable Broth (page 202)	4 cups finely shredded napa or savoy cabbage
1 tablespoon reduced-sodium soy sauce	6 flour tortillas
1 tablespoon Balsamic Vinegar	⅓ cup Plum Sauce (page 198)

Clean mushrooms and trim off stems.

Mix sesame oil, wine or broth, soy sauce, vinegar, and garlic in a large nonstick skillet. Heat until mixture bubbles, then add mushrooms, stem side up. Reduce heat to medium, cover and cook 3 minutes adding a small amount of water if the pan becomes dry.

Flip mushrooms, and cook second side until mushrooms are tender when pierced with a sharp knife, about 5 minutes. Remove from heat and cut mushrooms into ½-inch-wide strips.

Warm tortillas, one at a time, in a large, dry skillet, flipping to warm both sides until soft and pliable.

Lay several strips of mushroom on each tortilla. Top with strips of red pepper, shredded cabbage, and plum sauce. Wrap tortilla around filling and serve.

Per wrap: 155 calories; 5 g protein; 27 g carbohydrate;
4 g fat; 2 g fiber; 235 mg sodium; calories from protein: 13%;
calories from carbohydrates: 65%; calories from fats: 22%

SALADS

Three Sisters Salad
MAKES 8 1-CUP SERVINGS

Native Americans referred to squash, corn, and beans as the "three sisters" because they grow well together and their flavors and textures complement each other nicely in cooking.

2 cups butternut or kabocha squash, julienned or cut into 1/4-inch cubes
1 cup jicama, julienned or cut into 1/4-inch cubes
1 red bell pepper, seeded and diced
1 15-ounce can corn, drained
1 15-ounce can black beans, drained and rinsed

1/2 cup red onion, chopped
1/2 cup chopped cilantro
1/4 cup pumpkin seeds
1/4 cup seasoned rice vinegar
2 tablespoons lemon or lime juice
1 teaspoon cumin
1 teaspoon coriander
1 teaspoon chili powder
1 garlic clove, pressed or minced

Combine squash, jicama, bell pepper, corn, beans, onion, cilantro, and pumpkin seeds in a large bowl.

Mix vinegar, lemon juice, cumin, coriander, chili powder, and garlic. Pour over salad and toss to mix.

Per 1-cup serving: 170 calories; 8 g protein; 36 g carbohydrate;
1.4 g fat; 10 g fiber; 442 mg sodium; calories from protein: 17%;
calories from carbohydrates: 77%; calories from fats: 6%

* * *

Antipasto Salad
MAKES 6 1-CUP SERVINGS

The vegetables in this salad are steamed until they are just tender, then marinated in a vinaigrette dressing. This salad is delicious hot or cold.

1 large red potato, scrubbed
1 carrot, sliced
1 cup Italian green beans, fresh or frozen
1 cup cauliflower florets
1 small red bell pepper, seeded and sliced or diced
2 tablespoons finely chopped parsley
2 tablespoons balsamic vinegar

1 tablespoon seasoned rice vinegar
1 tablespoon olive oil
1 tablespoon lemon juice
2 teaspoons apple juice concentrate
2 garlic cloves, pressed
1 teaspoon stone-ground or Dijon-style mustard
¼ teaspoon salt
¼ teaspoon black pepper

Dice potatoes and steam with carrots over boiling water until just tender, about 10 minutes. Place in a salad bowl.

Steam green beans and cauliflower until just tender, 7 to 8 minutes. Add to salad bowl.

Add bell pepper and parsley.

In a small bowl, whisk together vinegars, oil, lemon juice, apple juice concentrate, garlic, mustard, salt, and pepper. Pour over vegetables and toss to mix.

Serve immediately or chill before serving.

Per 1-cup serving: 88 calories; 2 g protein; 16 g carbohydrate; 2 g fat; 2 g fiber; 212 mg sodium; calories from protein: 8%; calories from carbohydrates: 68%; calories from fats: 24%

● ● ●

Cucumber Salad

MAKES 3 1-CUP SERVINGS

This cool, crisp salad is perfect for hot summer days.

1 large cucumber, peeled
1 large tomato, diced
¼ cup finely chopped red onion
¼ cup chopped fresh basil or ½ teaspoon dried

3 tablespoons balsamic vinegar
¼ teaspoon salt
¼ teaspoon black pepper

Slice cucumbers in half lengthwise, scoop out seeds, then cut into bite-size pieces. Add remaining ingredients and toss to mix. Chill before serving.

Per 1-cup serving: 34 calories; 2 g protein; 8 g carbohydrate; 0.2 g fat; 2 g fiber; 186 mg sodium; calories from protein: 14%; calories from carbohydrates: 78%; calories from fats: 8%

● ● ●

Four Bean Salad

MAKES 10 1-CUP SERVINGS

This colorful salad is quick to prepare and keeps well.

1   15-ounce can dark kidney beans
1   15-ounce can vegetarian black-eyed peas
1   10-ounce package frozen lima beans, thawed
1   15-ounce can vegetarian chili beans
1   large red bell pepper, seeded and diced
½ cup finely chopped onion

2   cups corn, canned, frozen, or fresh
¼ cup seasoned rice vinegar
2   tablespoons apple cider or distilled vinegar
juice of 1 lemon
2   teaspoons cumin
1   teaspoon coriander
⅛ teaspoon cayenne

Drain kidney beans and black-eyed peas and place in a large bowl. Add lima beans, and chili beans with their sauce. Stir in bell pepper, onion, and corn.

Whisk together vinegars, lemon juice, cumin, coriander, and cayenne. Pour over salad and toss gently to mix. Chill at least 1 hour before serving, if possible.

Per 1-cup serving: 226 calories; 16 g protein; 40 g carbohydrate; 1.6 g fat; 10 g fiber; 434 mg sodium; calories from protein: 26%; calories from carbohydrates: 68%; calories from fats: 6%

● ● ●

Brown Rice Salad

MAKES ABOUT 16 ½-CUP SERVINGS

This salad is colorful and delicious. The addition of fruit adds interest and balance to this tasty and nutritious summer salad.

3   cups cooked Brown Rice (page 176)
3   green onions, chopped (about 1 cup)
½ green bell pepper, seeded and diced
½ red bell pepper, seeded and diced
1   stalk celery, thinly sliced
1   carrot, grated

1   green apple, cored and diced
1   cup finely shredded red cabbage
½ cup golden raisins
½ cup Tofu Mayo (page 201) or commercial vegan mayonnaise
3   tablespoons seasoned rice vinegar
2   teaspoons Dijon mustard
2   teaspoon curry powder

Place cooked rice in a large salad bowl.

Add onion, peppers, celery, carrot, apple, cabbage, and raisins.

Mix mayonnaise, vinegar, mustard, and curry powder. Pour over salad and toss to mix.

Per ½-cup serving: 211 calories; 4 g protein; 39 g carbohydrate;
5 g fat; 5 g fiber; 264 mg sodium; calories from protein: 8%;
calories from carbohydrates: 71%; calories from fats: 21%

● ● ●

Thai Noodle Salad
MAKES 8 1-CUP SERVINGS

This colorful salad is very filling. Udon is buckwheat pasta, similar to spaghetti, available in Asian markets, natural food stores, and some supermarkets. If you cannot find it, use spaghetti instead.

6 ounces udon or spaghetti
½ pound asparagus
1 red bell pepper, seeded and cut into 1-inch strips
3 green onions, thinly sliced
3 tablespoons peanut butter
3 tablespoons seasoned rice vinegar

2 teaspoons low-sodium soy sauce
1 teaspoon toasted sesame oil
2 teaspoons finely minced fresh ginger
1 large garlic clove, minced
⅛ teaspoon cayenne
1 cup fresh bean sprouts
½ cup chopped fresh cilantro

Cook pasta until just tender. Drain and rinse with cold water. Transfer to a salad bowl.

Snap tough ends off asparagus, then cut or break stalks into inch-long pieces. Bring a pot of water to a boil and add asparagus. Cook 1 minute. Drain and transfer to a bowl of ice water until chilled. Drain and add to pasta, along with bell pepper and green onions.

In a measuring cup or small bowl combine peanut butter, vinegar, soy sauce, sesame oil, ginger, garlic, and cayenne. Stir until smooth. Sauce should be pourable; if necessary, add a tablespoon or two of water. Pour over salad and toss to mix.

Top salad with bean sprouts and chopped cilantro.

Per 1-cup serving: 146 calories; 6 g protein; 23 g carbohydrate;
4 g fat; 4 g fiber; 252 mg sodium; calories from protein: 15%;
calories from carbohydrates: 61%; calories from fats: 24%

● ● ●

Lentil Salad
MAKES 8 1-CUP SERVINGS

This hearty salad can be a complete meal if you serve it on a bed of crisp romaine lettuce.

1 cup lentils
3 cups boiling water
3 cups cooked Brown Rice
   (page 176)
½ cup thinly sliced red onion
1 cucumber, peeled and sliced
2 tomatoes, diced
½ cup finely chopped parsley

⅓ to ½ cup lemon juice
1 tablespoon olive oil
1 tablespoon apple juice
   concentrate
1 garlic clove, pressed or minced
1 teaspoon paprika
½ teaspoon dry mustard
¾ teaspoon salt

Rinse lentils then add to a pan with boiling water. Cover loosely and simmer until just tender, about 25 minutes. Drain and transfer to a salad bowl. Cool.

When lentils are cool, add cooked rice, onion, cucumber, tomato, and parsley.

Whisk together lemon juice, olive oil, apple juice concentrate, garlic, paprika, dry mustard, and salt. Pour over salad and toss to mix.

Per 1-cup serving: 206 calories; 10 g protein; 38 g carbohydrate;
2 g fat; 4 g fiber; 210 mg sodium; calories from protein: 18%;
calories from carbohydrates: 70%; calories from fats: 12%

• • •

Spinach Salad with Curry Dressing
MAKES 8 1-CUP SERVINGS

This happy marriage of flavors and textures is especially easy to make if you use the prewashed spinach that is available in the produce departments of most supermarkets.

⅓ cup peanuts
1 tablespoon sesame seeds
1 bunch fresh spinach, washed, or
   1 6-ounce bag prewashed
   spinach (about 6 cups)
1 tart green apple, diced
2 green onions, thinly sliced,
   including green tops
¼ cup sultanas or golden raisins
3 tablespoons seasoned rice
   vinegar

3 tablespoons apple juice
   concentrate
2 teaspoons stone-ground or Dijon
   mustard
1 teaspoon reduced-sodium soy
   sauce
½ teaspoon curry powder
¼ teaspoon black pepper

Preheat oven to 375°F. Spread peanuts and sesame seeds in an oven-proof pan. Bake until lightly browned, about 10 minutes. Cool.

Combine spinach, apple, onions, and raisins in a large salad bowl. Add cooled peanuts and sesame seeds.

In a small bowl, whisk together vinegar, apple juice concentrate, mustard, soy sauce, curry powder, and black pepper.

Just before serving, pour dressing over salad and toss to mix.

Per 1-cup serving: 90 calories; 2 g protein; 14 g carbohydrate;
4 g fat; 2 g fiber; 272 mg sodium; calories from protein: 11%;
calories from carbohydrates: 56%; calories from fats: 33%

● ● ●

Tabouli
MAKES 6 1-CUP SERVINGS

A staple of Middle Eastern cuisines, Tabouli is often accompanied by stuffed grape leaves, or pita bread with hummus dip.

1   cup uncooked bulgur
2   cups boiling water
2   medium tomatoes, diced
3   green onions, chopped (about 1 cup)
½   cucumber, peeled and diced
½   cup finely chopped parsley
3   tablespoons finely chopped fresh mint leaves
juice of 1 or 2 lemons (about 3 to 5 tablespoons)
1   tablespoon olive oil
1   garlic clove, pressed or minced
½   teaspoon salt

Combine bulgur and boiling water in a mixing bowl. Cover and let stand until bulgur is tender, about 25 minutes. Drain off any excess liquid and use a fork to fluff bulgur. Cool.

When bulgur is cool, add tomatoes, green onions, cucumber, parsley, and mint. Whisk together lemon juice, oil, garlic, and salt. Add to bulgur mix and toss gently to mix. Chill before serving if time allows.

Per 1-cup serving: 120 calories; 4 g protein; 22 g carbohydrate;
2 g fat; 6 g fiber; 190 mg sodium; calories from protein: 12%;
calories from carbohydrates: 69%; calories from fats: 19%

DIPS, DRESSINGS, AND SAUCES

Red Pepper Hummus
MAKES ABOUT 2 CUPS

Red pepper hummus makes a delicious dip for fresh vegetables or pita wedges. It can also be used as a sandwich spread or as a filling in a wrap.

1   15-ounce can garbanzo beans, drained
½   cup water-packed roasted red pepper (about 2 peppers)
2   tablespoons tahini (sesame butter)
3   tablespoons lemon juice
1   garlic clove (or more to taste)
¼   teaspoon cumin

Combine drained beans, peppers, tahini, lemon juice, garlic, and cumin in a food processor. Process until completely smooth, about 2 minutes.

Per ¼ cup: 83 calories; 4 g protein; 13 g carbohydrate;
2 g fat; 2 g fiber; 70 mg sodium; calories from protein:
19%; calories from carbohydrates: 59%; calories from fats: 22%

● ● ●

Simple Vinaigrette
MAKES ½ CUP

Seasoned rice vinegar makes a delicious salad dressing all by itself, or enhanced with mustard and garlic.

½ cup seasoned rice vinegar
1 to 2 teaspoons stone-ground or
         Dijon-style mustard

1   clove garlic, pressed

Whisk all ingredients together. Use as a dressing for salads and for steamed vegetables.

Per tablespoon: 27 calories; 0.1 g protein; 6 g carbohydrate;
0.1 g fat; 0 g fiber; 562 mg sodium; calories from protein: 2%;
calories from carbohydrates: 94%; calories from fats: 4%

● ● ●

Balsamic Vinaigrette
MAKES ¼ CUP

The mellow flavor of balsamic vinegar is delicious on salads.

2   tablespoons balsamic vinegar
2   tablespoons seasoned rice
    vinegar

1   tablespoon ketchup
1   teaspoon stone-ground mustard
1   garlic clove, pressed

Whisk vinegars, ketchup, mustard, and garlic together.

Per tablespoon: 20 calories; 0.1 g protein; 4.5 g carbohydrate;
0.08 g fat; 0.05 g fiber; 229 mg sodium; calories from protein: 3%;
calories from carbohydrates: 93%; calories from fats: 4%

● ● ●

Piquant Dressing
MAKES ½ CUP

This dressing with a Mexican flavor can be as spicy as the salsa you use to make it.

¼ cup seasoned rice vinegar   1 garlic clove, pressed
¼ cup salsa

Whisk all ingredients together.

Per tablespoon: 3 calories; 0.02 g protein; 0.6 g carbohydrate;
0 g fat; 0.2 g fiber; 347 mg sodium; calories from protein: 3%;
calories from carbohydrates: 97%; calories from fats: 0%

• • •

Creamy Dill Dressing
MAKES ABOUT 1½ CUPS

This rich-tasting, creamy dressing has no added oil. Its creaminess comes from tofu.

1 12.3-ounce package Mori-Nu firm tofu
2 tablespoons lemon juice
3 tablespoons seasoned rice vinegar

1 tablespoon cider vinegar
1 teaspoon garlic granules or powder
½ teaspoon dill weed
¼ teaspoon salt

Combine all ingredients in a food processor or blender. Blend until completely smooth, 1 to 2 minutes. Store any extra dressing in an airtight container in the refrigerator.

Per tablespoon: 12 calories; 1 g protein; 1 g carbohydrate; 1 g fat;
0.1 g fiber; 90 mg sodium; calories from protein: 36%;
calories from carbohydrates: 18%; calories from fats: 46%

• • •

Salsa Fresca
MAKES ABOUT 6 CUPS

This fresh and chunky salsa is quite mild. For a hotter salsa, increase the jalapeños or red pepper flakes.

4 large ripe tomatoes, chopped (about 4 cups)
1 small onion, finely chopped
1 bell pepper, finely chopped
1 jalapeño pepper, seeded and finely chopped or 1 teaspoon red pepper flakes

4 garlic cloves, minced
1 cup chopped cilantro leaves
1 15-ounce can tomato sauce
2 tablespoons cider vinegar
1½ teaspoons cumin

Combine all ingredients in a mixing bowl. Stir to mix. Let stand 1 hour before serving.

Note: Salsa will keep in the refrigerator for about 2 weeks. It also freezes well.

Per tablespoon: 4 calories; 0.1 g protein; 1 g carbohydrate;
0.03 g fat; 0.2 g fiber; 27 mg sodium; calories from protein: 14%;
calories from carbohydrates: 79%; calories from fats: 7%

● ● ●

Apple Chutney
MAKES ABOUT 4 CUPS

Chutney is a spicy relish served as a condiment with Indian meals. This basic chutney is will keep in the refrigerator for several weeks, and may be frozen for longer storage.

3 large tart green apples (Granny Smith, pippin, or similar)
1 cup cider vinegar
1 cup sugar or other sweetener
1 large garlic clove, minced
1 tablespoon minced ginger root or ½ teaspoon powdered ginger

½ cup orange juice
1 teaspoon cinnamon
1 teaspoon powdered cloves
½ teaspoon salt
¼ teaspoon cayenne, or more to taste

Core apples and chop coarsely. Combine with vinegar, sugar, garlic, ginger root, orange juice, cinnamon, cloves, salt, and cayenne in a sauce pan

Bring to a slow simmer and cook uncovered, stirring occasionally, until most of the liquid is absorbed, about 1 hour.

Per tablespoon: 22 calories; 0.1 g protein; 6 g carbohydrate;
0.04 g fat; 0.2 g fiber; 17 mg sodium; calories from protein: 1%;
calories from carbohydrates: 97%; calories from fats: 2%

● ● ●

Plum Sauce
MAKES ABOUT 2 CUPS

Use this sauce as a condiment with curries.

1 17-ounce can purple plums in heavy syrup
2 garlic cloves
1 tablespoon cornstarch
2 tablespoons seasoned rice vinegar

1 tablespoon reduced-sodium soy sauce
⅛ teaspoon cayenne (more or less to taste)

Remove pits from plums. Place plums and their liquid, garlic, cornstarch, vinegar, soy sauce, and cayenne in a blender or food processor. Purée. Transfer to a saucepan and heat, stirring constantly, until thickened.

Per tablespoon: 17 calories; 0.1 g protein; 4 g carbohydrate;
0.01 g fat; 0.2 g fiber; 52 mg sodium; calories from protein: 2%;
calories from carbohydrates: 97%; calories from fats: 1%

• • •

Pineapple Apricot Sauce
MAKES ABOUT 3 CUPS

*Use this sauce as a spread on toast or as a topping for cake. It is delicious
with Quick and Easy Brown Bread (page 227). It is thickened with agar,
a sea vegetable thickener that is sold in natural food stores and Asian
markets.*

1 cup apple juice concentrate
1½ teaspoons agar powder
1 cup chopped apricots, fresh,
   frozen, or canned

1 8-ounce can crushed pineapple,
   packed in pineapple juice
¼ teaspoon ginger

Combine apple juice and agar with 1 cup water in a saucepan. Let stand
5 minutes. Bring to a simmer, stirring occasionally, and cook 3 minutes.
    Add apricots, pineapple with its juice, and ginger. Stir to mix. Remove
from heat and chill thoroughly, 3 to 4 hours.

Per tablespoon: 13 calories; 0.08 g protein; 3 g carbohydrate;
0 .05 g fat; 0.1 g fiber; 2 mg sodium; calories from protein: 3%;
calories from carbohydrates: 94%; calories from fats: 3%

• • •

Cool Cucumber Sauce
MAKES ABOUT 1½ CUPS

*Serve this cool creamy sauce with Instant Falafel Pockets (page 188) or
any other spicy foods.*

1 medium cucumber, peeled
1 12.3-ounce package Mori-Nu
   Lite Silken Tofu, firm or extra
   firm
2 tablespoons lemon juice

2 garlic cloves, pressed
¼ teaspoon salt
¼ teaspoon coriander
¼ teaspoon cumin

Cut cucumber in half, scoop out seeds, and and cut into chunks.
    Place cucumber, tofu, lemon juice, garlic, salt, and spices in food
processor and purée until completely smooth, about 3 minutes.

Per tablespoon: 8 calories; 1 g protein; g carbohydrate;
0.4 g fat; 0.2 g fiber; 23 mg sodium; calories from protein: 35%;
calories from carbohydrates: 21%; calories from fats: 44%

• • •

Sesame Salt
MAKES ½ CUP

Sesame Salt is a delicious alternative to butter or margarine on cooked grains, baked potatoes, or steamed vegetables. Unhulled sesame seeds (sometimes called "brown sesame seeds") are sold in natural food stores and some supermarkets.

½ cup unhulled sesame seeds   ½ teaspoon salt

Toast sesame seeds in a dry skillet over medium heat, stirring constantly until they begin to pop and brown slightly, about 5 minutes. Transfer to a blender. Add salt and grind into a uniform powder. Transfer to an airtight container. Store in refrigerator.

Per tablespoon: 52 calories; 2 g protein; 2 g carbohydrate;
4 g fat; 1 g fiber; 134 mg sodium; calories from protein: 12%;
calories from carbohydrates: 15%; calories from fats: 73%

● ● ●

Sesame Seasoning
MAKES ½ CUP

Sesame Seasoning is delicious with steamed vegetables, cooked grains, and legumes. Unhulled sesame seeds are light brown in color and are sold in natural food stores and some supermarkets.

½ cup unhulled sesame seeds   2 tablespoons nutritional yeast
½ teaspoon salt

Toast sesame seeds in a dry skillet over medium heat. Stir constantly until seeds begin to pop and brown slightly, about 5 minutes.

Transfer to a blender, add salt and nutritional yeast and grind into a fine powder.

Transfer to an airtight container. Store in refrigerator.

Per tablespoon: 57 calories; 2 g protein; 3 g carbohydrate;
4 g fat; 1 g fiber; 137 mg sodium; calories from protein: 15%;
calories from carbohydrates: 19%; calories from fats: 66%

● ● ●

Tofu Mayo
MAKES ABOUT 1½ CUPS

Use this low-fat mayonnaise substitute on sandwiches and salads.

1 12.3-ounce package Mori-Nu
   Lite Silken Tofu (firm or extra
   firm)
¾ teaspoon salt
½ teaspoon sugar

1 teaspoon Dijon mustard
1½ tablespoons lemon juice
1½ tablespoons seasoned rice
   vinegar

Combine tofu, salt, sugar, mustard, lemon juice and vinegar in a food processor or blender, and process until completely smooth, 1 to 2 minutes. Chill thoroughly before using.

Per tablespoon: 6 calories; 1 g protein; 0.4 g carbohydrate;
0.1 g fat; 0 g fiber; 93 mg sodium; calories from protein: 48%;
calories from carbohydrates: 29%; calories from fats: 23%

* * *

Corn Butter
MAKES ABOUT 2 CUPS

This creamy yellow spread is a low-fat alternative to margarine. Emes Jel and agar powder are thickening agents that are sold in natural food stores.

¼ cup cornmeal
2 teaspoons Emes Jel (see
   Glossary) or 1½ teaspoons agar
   powder
1 cup boiling water
2 tablespoons raw cashews

½ teaspoon salt
2 teaspoons lemon juice
1 tablespoon finely grated raw
   carrot
1 teaspoon nutritional yeast
   (optional)

Combine cornmeal with 1 cup water in a small saucepan. Simmer, stirring frequently, until very thick, about 10 minutes. Set aside.

Combine Emes Jel or agar powder with ¼ cup cold water in a blender. Let stand at least 3 minutes. Add 1 cup boiling water and blend to mix. Add cooked cornmeal, cashews, salt, lemon juice, grated carrot, and yeast, if using. Cover and blend until totally smooth (this is essential and will take several minutes). Transfer to a covered container and chill until thickened, 2 to 3 hours.

Per tablespoon: 7 calories; 0.2 g protein; 1 g carbohydrate;
0.2 g fat; 0.1 g fiber; 34 mg sodium; calories from protein: 11%;
calories from carbohydrates: 57%; calories from fats: 32%

* * *

Brown Gravy

MAKES ABOUT 2 CUPS

This traditional-tasting gravy is low in fat and delicious on potatoes, rice, or vegetables.

2 cups water or vegetable broth
1 tablespoon cashews
1 tablespoon onion powder
½ teaspoon garlic granules or powder

2 tablespoons cornstarch
3 tablespoons reduced-sodium soy sauce

Combine all ingredients in blender container. Blend until completely smooth, 2 to 3 minutes.

Transfer to a saucepan and cook over medium heat, stirring constantly, until thickened.

Per ¼-cup serving: 23 calories; 1 g protein; 4 g carbohydrate;
0.5 g fat; 0.1 g fiber; 190 mg sodium; calories from protein: 15%;
calories from carbohydrates: 65%; calories from fats: 20%

* * *

SOUPS AND STEWS

Vegetable Broth

MAKES ABOUT 2 QUARTS

A steamy cup of this broth makes a warm and comforting meal. It may also be used as an ingredient in recipes that call for broth or stock.

1 onion, chopped
1 carrot, chopped
1 celery stalk, chopped
¼ cup chopped fresh parsley
6 cups water
2 teaspoons onion powder
½ teaspoon thyme

¼ teaspoon turmeric
¼ teaspoon garlic powder
¼ teaspoon marjoram
½ teaspoon salt
1 15-ounce can garbanzo beans, including liquid

Combine onion, carrot, celery, parsley, water, onion powder, thyme, turmeric, garlic powder, and marjoram in a large pot. Cover and simmer 20 minutes.

Stir in garbanzo beans with their liquid. Transfer to a blender in small batches and process until completely smooth, about 1 minute per batch. Be sure to hold the lid on tightly and start the blender on the lowest speed.

Per 1-cup serving: 80 calories; 3 g protein; 16 g carbohydrate;
1 g fat; 3 g fiber; 302 mg sodium; calories from protein: 15%;
calories from carbohydrates: 77%; calories from fats: 8%

* * *

African Bean Soup

MAKES 8 1-CUP SERVINGS

Sweet potatoes and peanuts are familiar ingredients in many African cuisines. In this colorful soup they are combined with garbanzo beans and other vegetables and served over cooked rice.

3 tablespoons reduced-sodium soy sauce
1 onion, sliced
2 small sweet potatoes or yams, peeled and diced (about 2 cups)
1 large carrot, thinly sliced
1 celery stalk, thinly sliced
1 red bell pepper, seeded and diced

1 15-ounce can crushed tomatoes
1 quart Vegetable Broth (page 202) or water
1 15-ounce can garbanzo beans
½ cup chopped fresh cilantro
3 tablespoons peanut butter
1 to 2 teaspoons curry powder
cooked brown rice

Heat ½ cup water and soy sauce in a large pot. Add onion and sweet potatoes and cook over high heat, stirring often, until onion is soft, about 5 minutes.

Add carrot, celery, and pepper. Cover and cook 3 minutes, stirring occasionally.

Add tomatoes, vegetable broth, garbanzo beans and their liquid, cilantro, peanut butter, and curry powder. Stir to mix, then cover and simmer until vegetables are fork tender, about 10 minutes.

To serve, place about ½ cup of cooked brown rice in a bowl and top it with a generous ladle of soup.

Per 1-cup soup over ½-cup rice: 257 calories;
8 g protein; 47 g carbohydrate; 5 g fat; 6 g fiber; 432 mg sodium;
calories from protein: 13%; calories from carbohydrates:
70%; calories from fats: 17%

* * *

Portuguese Kale Soup

MAKES 12 1-CUP SERVINGS

This hearty soup is a delicious way to enjoy calcium-rich kale. Yves Veggie Breakfast Links are sold in natural food stores and many supermarkets.

1 tablespoon olive oil
1 onion, chopped
1 large carrot, scrubbed and diced
2 celery stalks, thinly sliced
2 russet potatoes, scrubbed and diced
3 garlic cloves, minced
2 teaspoons dried oregano

1 teaspoon dried basil
¼ teaspoon black pepper
¼ teaspoon salt
1 15-ounce can cannelini beans
4 cups Vegetable Broth (page 202)
½ pound kale
1 7-ounce package Yves Veggie Breakfast Links

Heat oil in a large pot and add onion, carrot, and celery. Cook over high heat, stirring often, until onions are soft, about 5 minutes.

Reduce heat to medium and stir in potatoes, garlic, oregano, basil, pepper, and salt. Add ¼ cup water, then cover and cook, stirring often, 5 minutes.

Stir in cannelini beans and their liquid, and vegetable broth. Cover and simmer until potatoes are just tender, about 10 minutes.

Remove stems from kale and chop leaves into small pieces. Add to soup.

Cut Breakfast Links into bite-size chunks and add to soup. Cover and simmer until kale is tender, about 5 minutes.

Per 1-cup serving: 127 calories; 9 g protein; 22 g carbohydrate;
2 g fat; 5 g fiber; 399 mg sodium; calories from protein: 26%;
calories from carbohydrates: 62%; calories from fats: 12%

* * *

Chili Potato Soup
MAKES 10 1-CUP SERVINGS

Chilies add a spicy interest to traditional potato soup.

4 russet potatoes
1 tablespoon olive oil
1 large onion, chopped
2 cloves garlic, minced
1 large bell pepper, seeded and finely diced
1 cup chopped cilantro (optional)
1 teaspoon cumin
1 teaspoon basil

¼ teaspoon black pepper
1 4-ounce can diced Anaheim chilies
2 cups unsweetened fortified soy milk or rice milk
½ to 1 teaspoon salt
2 green onions, finely chopped, including tops

Peel potatoes and cut into ½-inch cubes. Place in a large pot with just enough water to cover. Cover and simmer until tender, about 20 minutes.

While potatoes cook, heat oil in a large skillet and cook onion 2 minutes. Add garlic, bell pepper, cilantro if using, cumin, basil, and black pepper. Cook over medium-high heat, stirring often, until onion is soft, about 3 minutes.

When potatoes are tender, mash them in their water. Add onion mixture, along with diced chilies, and milk. Add salt to taste. Stir to blend, then heat gently until steamy. Sprinkle with chopped green onions and serve.

Per 1-cup serving: 127 calories; 3 g protein; 27 g carbohydrate;
2 g fat; 3 g fiber; 248–496 mg sodium; calories from protein: 9%;
calories from carbohydrates: 78%; calories from fats: 13%

● ● ●

Borscht
MAKES 8 1-CUP SERVINGS

This delicious vegetable soup can be eaten plain, or with the optional creamy topping. Serve it with rye bread and a crisp green salad.

1 to 2 beets, peeled and diced
    (about 1 cup)
1 small onion chopped
1 medium potato, cut in $1/4$-inch cubes
1 carrot, sliced or diced
1 celery stalk, thinly sliced
1 cup finely shredded green cabbage

4 cups Vegetable Broth (page 202)
1 cup crushed tomatoes
$1/2$ teaspoon dill weed
$1/2$ teaspoon caraway seeds
$1/8$ teaspoon black pepper

Optional Topping:
$1/2$ cup Tofu Mayo (page 201)
5 tablespoons lemon juice

Combine beets, onion, potato, carrot, celery, cabbage, Vegetable Broth, tomatoes, dill weed, caraway seeds, and black pepper in a large pot. Bring to a simmer, then cover and cook until beets and potatoes are tender, about 25 minutes.

For topping, mix Tofu Mayo and lemon juice.

Ladle soup into bowls and garnish with 1 to 2 tablespoons of topping.

Per 1-cup serving (with topping): 80 calories; 4 g protein;
16 g carbohydrate; 1 g fat; 2.5 g fiber; 372 mg sodium;
calories from protein: 16%; calories from carbohydrates:
73%; calories from fats: 11%

Per 1-cup serving (without topping): 66 calories; 2 g protein;
14 g carbohydrate; 0.3 g fat; 2 g fiber; 302 mg sodium;
calories from protein: 14%; calories from carbohydrates:
82%; calories from fats: 4%

● ● ●

Black Bean Soup

MAKES 8 1-CUP SERVINGS

This smooth and creamy soup is a perfect make-ahead meal because it's even better the second day. Serve it with whole grain bread and a fresh vegetable salad.

1 cup dry black beans	2 bay leaves
1 tablespoon olive oil	1 teaspoon oregano
1 onion, chopped	¼ teaspoon savory
2 stalks celery, chopped	⅛ teaspoon black pepper
1 large carrot, chopped	2 tablespoons lemon juice
1 potato, diced	2 tablespoons red wine (optional)
2 large garlic cloves, pressed	1 teaspoon salt
6 cups Vegetable Broth (page 202) or water	

Rinse beans, then soak in about 5 cups of water for 6 to 8 hours or overnight. Drain and rinse.

In a large pot heat oil and cook onion until soft, stirring often, about 5 minutes. Add celery, carrot, potato, garlic, and ¼ cup water. Cook over medium heat 3 minutes, stirring constantly.

Add Vegetable Broth, soaked beans, bay leaves, oregano, savory, and black pepper. Cover and simmer until beans are very soft, stirring occasionally, about 1 hour.

Remove bay leaves. Puree in small batches in a blender until very smooth. Be sure to start on low speed and hold the lid on tightly. Pour soup back into pan and stir in lemon juice, wine if using, and salt. Heat until steamy.

Crock-Pot Version: Clean and soak beans as above. Place all ingredients except lemon juice and salt into a crockpot. Cover and cook on high until beans are tender, about 3 hours if you start with boiling water, 6 to 8 hours if you start with cold water. Remove bay leaves and proceed as directed above.

Per 1-cup serving: 86 calories; 3 g protein; 16 g carbohydrate;
1 g fat; 3.5 g fiber; 286 mg sodium; calories from protein: 14%;
calories from carbohydrates: 74%; calories from fats: 12%

● ● ●

Black-Eyed Pea Stew

MAKES 8 1-CUP SERVINGS

For a delicious down-home meal, serve this easy-to-prepare stew with Braised Collards or Kale (page 219).

1½ cups dried black-eyed peas
2 teaspoons olive oil
2 onions, chopped
4 garlic cloves, minced
2 celery stalks, sliced
½ cup short-grain brown rice

1 bunch cilantro, chopped
½ teaspoon red pepper flakes
4 cups Vegetable Broth (page 202)
½ teaspoon salt
Sesame Salt (page 200)

Rinse black-eyed peas, then soak overnight in at least 6 cups cold water.

Gently heat olive oil in a large pot, then add chopped onions, garlic, and celery. Cook over high heat, stirring often, until onion is soft, about 5 minutes. Add a tablespoon or two of water if the mixture begins to stick.

Drain soaked black-eyed peas and add to the pot along with rice, cilantro, pepper flakes, and Vegetable Broth. Cover and simmer until beans and rice are tender, about 45 minutes. Add salt to taste.

To serve, ladle some stew into a bowl and sprinkle with a teaspoon of Sesame Salt.

Per 1-cup serving: 184 calories; 9 g protein; 34 g carbohydrate;
2 g fat; 5 g fiber; 284 mg sodium; calories from protein: 20%;
calories from carbohydrates: 71%; calories from fats: 9%

• • •

Cream of Asparagus Soup
MAKES 7 1-CUP SERVINGS

2 medium potatoes
1 bunch fresh asparagus
2 cups shredded cabbage
1 cup loosely packed chopped
  parsley

¼ cup chopped fresh basil
1 to 2 cups unsweetened fortified
  soy milk or rice milk
¾ teaspoon salt

Scrub and dice potatoes (no need to peel them). Place in a large pot with 2 cups of water. Bring to a simmer, then cover and cook until tender when pierced with a fork, about 10 minutes.

Remove tough ends from asparagus, then cut or break it into 1-inch lengths; you should have about 4 cups.

When potatoes are tender, add asparagus along with cabbage, parsley, and basil. Cover and simmer until asparagus is just tender, about 5 minutes.

Use a blender to puree vegetables in 2 or 3 batches, adding some of the milk to each batch. Be sure to start blender on a low speed and hold lid on tightly. Return soup to pan, add salt to taste, then heat until steamy.

Per 1-cup serving: 101 calories; 4 g protein; 21 g carbohydrate;
1 g fat; 4 g fiber; 243 mg sodium; calories from protein: 16%;
calories from carbohydrates: 79%; calories from fats: 5%

ENTRÉES

Mexican Skillet Pie

MAKES 12 SERVINGS

This stovetop entrée requires a very large skillet (14-inch or larger). If you don't have a skillet this large, you can assemble it in a 9-by-13-inch baking dish and bake it at 350°F for 30 minutes.

1 15-ounce can garbanzo beans, drained
1½ cups water-packed roasted red peppers (about 6 peppers), divided
2 garlic cloves, peeled
1 tablespoon tahini (sesame butter)
3 tablespoons lemon juice
½ teaspoon cumin

1 onion, chopped
4 garlic cloves, minced
1 28-ounce can crushed tomatoes
12 corn tortillas
2 15-ounce cans vegetarian chili beans
1 15-ounce can corn kernels, drained
3 green onions, chopped

Combine garbanzo beans, 2 of the roasted peppers, garlic, tahini, lemon juice, and cumin in a food processor or blender and process until completely smooth, 2 to 3 minutes. Set aside.

Heat ½ cup water in a 14-inch or larger skillet. Add onion and garlic and cook over high heat for five minutes, stirring occasionally. Stir in crushed tomatoes, then arrange tortillas on top (there will be several layers).

Spread chili beans evenly over tortillas and top with the remaining roasted red peppers, drained corn, and an even layer of the garbanzo mixture.

Cover skillet and cook over medium heat until hot and steamy, 15 to 20 minutes. Sprinkle with chopped green onions and serve.

Per serving (¹⁄₁₂th of pie): 257 calories; 18 g protein; 42 g carbohydrate; 4 g fat; 7 g fiber; 459 mg sodium; calories from protein: 27%; alories from carbohydrates: 61%; calories from fats: 12%

⬤ ⬤ ⬤

Red Lentil Curry

MAKES 6 ½-CUP SERVINGS

This curry is made with small, brightly colored lentils called masoor *dal that are sold in natural food stores, ethnic markets, and some supermarkets. They are ideal for quick meals as they cook in just 20 minutes. If you are not able to locate these lentils, yellow split peas may be substituted in this recipe.*

1 cup red lentils	$\frac{1}{2}$ teaspoon turmeric
$\frac{1}{2}$ teaspoon salt	$\frac{1}{2}$ teaspoon cumin
3 cups boiling water	$\frac{1}{2}$ teaspoon coriander
1 tablespoon olive oil	$\frac{1}{4}$ teaspoon ginger
1 teaspoon mustard seeds	$\frac{1}{8}$ teaspoon cayenne

Rinse lentils and place in a pot with salt and boiling water. Cover loosely and simmer until completely tender, 15 to 20 minutes (45 minutes for yellow split peas).

In a large skillet, heat oil and add mustard seeds, turmeric, cumin, coriander, ginger, and cayenne. Cook over medium heat, stirring constantly, until mustard seeds begin to pop, about 1 minute. Be careful not to inhale the fumes, as these can be irritating.

Remove skillet from heat and add cooked lentils slowly and carefully to keep them from splattering. Return skillet to heat and simmer gently, stirring occasionally until lentils are the consistency of refried beans, about 15 minutes.

Per $\frac{1}{2}$-cup serving: 128 calories; 9 g protein; 18 g carbohydrate;
3 g fat; 4 g fiber; 181 mg sodium; calories from protein: 28%;
calories from carbohydrates: 55%; calories from fats: 17%

● ● ●

Spicy Indian Garbanzos
MAKES 8 $\frac{1}{2}$-CUP SERVINGS

Serve over cooked rice and top with a spoonful of Apple Chutney (page 198).

2 teaspoons toasted sesame oil	$\frac{1}{2}$ teaspoon turmeric
1 onion, chopped	$\frac{1}{2}$ teaspoon coriander
1 tablespoon fresh chopped ginger	$\frac{1}{2}$ teaspoon cinnamon
1 tablespoon chopped garlic	$\frac{1}{2}$ teaspoon cumin
2 15-ounce cans garbanzo beans	$\frac{1}{2}$ teaspoon black pepper
$\frac{1}{2}$ cup chopped cilantro (optional)	$\frac{1}{2}$ teaspoon salt

Heat oil in a large nonstick skillet or pot. Cook onion over high heat for 3 minutes, then stir in ginger and garlic. Reduce heat to medium-high and cook, stirring often, until onion is soft, about 3 minutes.

Stir in garbanzo beans and their liquid, cilantro, turmeric, coriander, cinnamon, cumin, and black pepper. Cover and cook, stirring occasionally, 15 minutes. Stir in salt.

To serve, place a portion of cooked rice on each plate. Top with an equal amount of the garbanzo mixture and a spoonful of Apple Chutney.

Per ½-cup serving: 156 calories; 6 g protein; 27 g carbohydrate; 3 g fat;
5 g fiber; 453 mg sodium; calories from protein: 14%; calories from
carbohydrates: 69%; calories from fats: 17%

● ● ●

Broccoli and Bok Choy with Baked Tofu
MAKES 6 1-CUP SERVINGS

*This simple recipe is a delicious way to add healthful greens and soy to
your diet. Serve with Brown Rice (page 176), pasta, or Grilled Polenta
(page 181).*

2 teaspoons olive oil
1 small onion, finely chopped
2 cups broccoli florets
3 to 4 cups thinly sliced, bok choy
4 ounces baked tofu, cut into
   ½-inch cubes

¼ teaspoon black pepper
2 to 3 teaspoons reduced-sodium
   soy sauce
brown rice, pasta, or polenta for
   serving

Heat oil in a large nonstick skillet, then add onion and cook over high
heat, stirring often, 2 to 3 minutes.

Add broccoli and bok choy and continue cooking, stirring constantly,
for 2 minutes.

Stir in 2 tablespoons water, along with tofu, black pepper, and soy
sauce. Cover and cook until broccoli and bok choy are just tender and tofu
is heated through, about 3 minutes.

Per 1-cup serving (with 1 cup brown rice): 287 calories;
10.5 g protein; 51 g carbohydrate; 5 g fat; 2 g fiber;
220 mg sodium; calories from protein: 14%;
calories from carbohydrates: 70%; calories from fats: 16%

● ● ●

Sweet and Sour Stir-Fry
MAKES 8 1-CUP SERVINGS

*This colorful stir-fry is made with seitan, a high-protein, meatlike ingre-
dient made from wheat. Look for it in the refrigerated section of your
favorite natural food store.*

⅓ cup ketchup
⅓ cup cider vinegar
⅓ cup brown sugar
2 tablespoons reduced-sodium soy
   sauce
1 tablespoon cornstarch

¼ teaspoon dried red pepper flakes
2 teaspoons toasted sesame oil
1 cup thinly sliced onion
2 cups sliced mushrooms
1 8-ounce package of seitan, cut
   into strips

1   red bell pepper, seeded and
    thinly sliced
1   medium zucchini, thinly sliced

2   cups snow peas
8   cups cooked basmati or jasmine
    rice

Combine ketchup, vinegar, sugar, soy sauce, cornstarch, pepper flakes, and ½ cup water in a small bowl. Stir to mix, then set aside.

In a large skillet or wok, heat sesame oil and add onion slices. Cook over high heat, stirring often, until onion begins to soften, about 3 minutes. Add mushrooms and cook 3 minutes

Add seitan strips to mushrooms along with bell pepper, zucchini, and snow peas. Cook over medium-high heat, stirring constantly, until vegetables are just barely tender, about 3 minutes. Add reserved sauce mixture and cook, stirring constantly until sauce is clear and thickened, about 2 minutes. Serve over cooked rice.

Per 1-cup serving with 1 cup rice: 334 calories; 14 g protein; 63 g carbohydrate; 3 g fat; 5 g fiber; 326 mg sodium; calories from protein: 17%; calories from carbohydrates: 75%; calories from fats: 8%

● ● ●

Black Bean Hash

MAKES ABOUT 6 1-CUP SERVINGS

Serve this colorful hash for a hearty breakfast or a satisfying dinner. For a take-along meal, roll it in a flour tortilla.

2   teaspoons olive oil
1   onion, chopped or sliced
3   garlic cloves, minced
1   large red potato, cut into ¼-inch
    dice
1   small green bell pepper, seeded
    and diced
1   cup chopped tomatoes, fresh or
    canned

1   tablespoon chili powder
¼   teaspoon cumin
1   15-ounce can black beans,
    drained and rinsed
1   cup frozen corn
¼ to ½ teaspoon salt

Heat oil in a large skillet. Add onion, garlic, and potato. Cook, stirring frequently, for 3 minutes.

Add bell pepper, tomatoes, chili powder, cumin, and ¾ cup water. Cover and simmer until potatoes are soft, about 10 minutes.

Stir in beans and corn. Add salt to taste.

Per 1-cup serving: 152 calories; 6 g protein; 29 g carbohydrate; 2 g fat; 6 g fiber; 315 mg sodium; calories from protein: 16%; calories from carbohydrates: 72%; calories from fats: 12%

● ● ●

Simple Pasta Supper

MAKES 8 1-CUP SERVINGS

Calcium-rich kale and kidney beans offer this garlicky meal added nutritional punch. Serve with a tossed green salad and whole grain bread for dinner on a busy night.

8 ounces pasta spirals	1 15-ounce can red kidney beans
1 tablespoon olive oil	2 cups finely chopped fresh kale
1 onion chopped	½ cup chopped fresh basil
6 large garlic cloves, chopped	¼ teaspoon black pepper
1 cup vegetable juice (V-8 juice, Very Veggie, or similar)	

Cook pasta until tender, then rinse and drain. Set aside.

Heat oil in a large pot. Add onion and garlic and cook over medium heat, stirring often, until onion begins to brown, about 10 minutes.

Stir in juice, scraping pan to remove any stuck bits of onion, then add kidney beans with their liquid, kale, basil, and black pepper. Stir to mix, then cover and simmer, stirring occasionally, until kale is tender, about 5 minutes.

Per 1-cup serving: 195 calories; 8 g protein; 36 g carbohydrate; 2 g fat; 8 g fiber; 208 mg sodium; calories from protein: 16%; calories from carbohydrates: 73%; calories from fats: 11%

● ● ●

Polenta Pizza

MAKES 12 SERVINGS

Although this recipe involves some extra effort, it is not difficult and the results are well worth it.

5 cups water	3 teaspoons basil, divided
1 cup polenta	1 pound firm tofu
½ teaspoon salt	1½ tablespoons white miso
½ teaspoon thyme	1 tablespoon tahini (sesame butter)
½ teaspoon oregano	¼ cup water
10 sun-dried tomato halves	3 or 4 garlic cloves, minced
½ cup boiling water	2 10-ounce packages frozen chopped spinach, thawed
1 large onion, finely chopped	
6 large garlic cloves	2 teaspoons balsamic vinegar
½ pound mushrooms, chopped	1 tablespoon reduced-sodium soy sauce
12 ounces roasted red peppers, finely chopped	
1 cup tomato sauce	⅛ teaspoon black pepper

Whisk polenta into water, then add salt, thyme, and oregano. Simmer over medium heat, stirring often, until very thick, about 25 minutes. Spread in an even layer, about ¼-inch thick, on a large baking sheet. Cool.

Soak sun-dried tomatoes in boiling water until soft, about 10 minutes. Chop and set aside.

Heat ½ cup water and cook onions, garlic, and mushrooms until soft, about 5 minutes. Add chopped tomatoes, roasted red peppers, and 1 teaspoon basil. Simmer 5 minutes.

Place tofu in a clean dish towel and squeeze to remove some of the water. Transfer to a food processor. Add miso, 2 teaspoons basil, and tahini. Process until completely smooth.

Heat ¼ cup water in a large skillet, then add garlic. Cook 1 minute, then add spinach, vinegar, soy sauce, and pepper. Cook, stirring often, until all the liquid is evaporated.

Preheat oven to 350°F.

To assemble pizza: spread tofu mixture evenly over polenta. Top with spinach, then sprinkle with tomato sauce. Bake for 20 minutes.

Per slice (¹⁄₁₂th of pizza): 127 calories; 7 g protein; 20 g carbohydrate; 3 g fat; 4 g fiber; 376 mg sodium; calories from protein: 22%; calories from carbohydrates: 58%; calories from fats: 20%

● ● ●

Shepherd's Pie
MAKES 12 SERVINGS

This is a hearty vegetable casserole topped with a delicious mashed potato crust.

2 onions, chopped	4 russet potatoes, peeled and diced
1 bell pepper, seeded and diced	1 cup unsweetened fortified soy
2 carrots, sliced	milk or rice milk
2 stalks of celery, sliced	¼ teaspoon onion powder
2½ cups sliced mushrooms (about	¼ teaspoon garlic powder
½ pound)	½ teaspoon salt
1 15-ounce can crushed or ground	1½ tablespoons rice flour
tomatoes	2 tablespoons potato flour
1 15-ounce can kidney beans,	½ cup Corn Butter (page 201) or
drained	1 tablespoon nonhydrogenated
½ teaspoon paprika	margarine
½ teaspoon black pepper	additional paprika for sprinkling on
2 tablespoons reduced-sodium soy	potatoes
sauce	

Heat ½ cup water in a large pot and add onions. Cook over high heat, stirring occasionally, for 3 minutes.

Add bell pepper, carrots, and celery. Reduce heat slightly and cook 5 minutes, stirring occasionally.

Add mushrooms, then cover pan and cook 7 minutes, stirring occasionally.

Add tomatoes, kidney beans, paprika, black pepper, and soy sauce. Cover and cook 15 minutes.

In the meantime, steam potatoes over boiling water until tender when pierced with a fork, about 15 minutes. Transfer to a bowl and mash.

Pour milk into a blender and add onion powder, garlic powder, salt, rice flour, potato flour, and Corn Butter or margarine. Blend until completely smooth, 1 to 2 minutes, then add to mashed potatoes and mix well.

Preheat oven to 350°F.

Transfer vegetables to a 9-by-13-inch baking dish. Spread mashed potatoes evenly over top. Sprinkle with paprika.

Bake for 25 minutes, until hot and bubbly.

Per serving (¹⁄₁₂th of casserole made with Corn Butter): 178 calories; 7 g protein; 37 g carbohydrate; 1 g fat; 7 g fiber; 271 mg sodium; calories from protein: 15%; calories from carbohydrates: 80%; calories from fats: 5%

Per serving (¹⁄₁₂th of casserole made with margarine): 182 calories; 7 g protein; 36 g carbohydrate; 2 g fat; 7 g fiber; 257 mg sodium; calories from protein: 14%; calories from carbohydrates: 77%; calories from fats: 9%

* * *

Hearty Barbecue Beans

MAKES 8 1-CUP SERVINGS

These spicy beans are a great accompaniment to meatless hot dogs (page 186).

1 16-ounce can Vegetarian Baked Beans	1 cup finely chopped onion
1 15-ounce can kidney beans	1 tablespoon cider vinegar
1 10-ounce package frozen baby lima beans	1 tablespoon molasses
1 cup crushed tomatoes	2 teaspoons stone-ground mustard
	1 teaspoon chili powder

Combine all ingredients in a pot. Cover and simmer, stirring occasionally, for 25 to 30 minutes.

Per 1-cup serving: 168 calories; 9 g protein; 34 g carbohydrate; 1 g fat; 9 g fiber; 493 mg sodium; calories from protein: 20%; calories from carbohydrates: 77%; calories from fats: 3%

* * *

Pan-seared Portobello Mushrooms

MAKES 4 SERVINGS

These giant mushrooms make a hearty, meatlike entree. Serve them with brown rice, pasta, or couscous.

4 large portobello mushrooms
2 teaspoons olive oil
2 tablespoons red wine or water
2 tablespoons reduced-sodium soy sauce

1 tablespoon balsamic vinegar
2 garlic cloves, pressed
½ teaspoon oregano

Clean mushrooms, trimming stems flush with bottom of caps.

Mix oil, wine or water, soy sauce, vinegar, garlic, and oregano in a large skillet. Heat until mixture begins to bubble, then add mushrooms, top side down. Reduce to medium heat, cover and cook 3 minutes. (If the pan becomes dry, add 2 to 3 tablespoons of water). Turn mushrooms and cook second side until tender when pierced with a sharp knife, about 5 minutes. Serve hot.

Per mushroom: 63 calories; 3 g protein; 7 g carbohydrate;
3 g fat; 2 g fiber; 258 mg sodium; calories from protein: 20%;
calories from carbohydrates: 43%; calories from fats: 37%

● ● ●

Tofu Brochettes

MAKES 8 BROCHETTES

Enjoy these brochettes at your next family barbecue or cook them indoors under the boiler. The tofu should marinate for several hours before cooking, so this is a perfect make-ahead dish. Serve them with cooked Brown Rice (page 176) or Grilled Polenta (page 181).

1 pound very firm tofu
1 teaspoon oregano
1 teaspoon thyme
¼ cup reduced-sodium soy sauce
2 tablespoons balsamic vinegar
2 tablespoons red wine or additional balsamic vinegar
2 garlic cloves, crushed

¼ teaspoon black pepper
8 cherry tomatoes
1 small red onion
½ green bell pepper
½ red bell pepper
16 button mushrooms
2 small zucchini

Line a baking sheet with a clean dish towel. Cut tofu into 1-inch thick slices and place on the dish towel in a single layer. Cover with a second clean dish towel and a cutting board. Place several heavy objects (canned food, books, jars of beans) on the cutting board. Let stand 30 minutes.

In the meantime, prepare marinade. Toast oregano and thyme in a dry skillet over medium-low heat, stirring constantly, for 1 minute. Remove from heat. Let pan cool then stir in soy sauce, vinegar, wine, garlic, and black pepper.

Cut tofu slices into 1-inch cubes and place into a zip-top plastic bag. Add marinade and seal the bag, then gently turn it so that all tofu pieces are coated with marinade. Refrigerate 4 hours or more (overnight is ideal), turning the bag occasionally to keep tofu evenly coated.

To prepare vegetables, stem tomatoes, cut onion into ½-inch chunks, cut peppers into 1-inch pieces, clean mushrooms, and slice zucchini into ¼-inch thick rounds.

To assemble brochettes, arrange an assortment of vegetables and marinated tofu onto skewers.

Preheat grill or broiler, then cook brochettes, turning every few minutes to expose all sides to the heat until vegetables are lightly browned, 5 to 10 minutes.

Per brochette: 71 calories; 6 g protein; 6 g carbohydrate; 3 g fat;
2 g fiber; 134 mg sodium; calories from protein: 32%;
calories from carbohydrates: 34%; calories from fats: 34%

* * *

Macaroni with Creamy Tofu Sauce
MAKES 8 1-CUP SERVINGS

Here's a healthy version of a traditional "comfort food."

8 ounces eggless macaroni
1 tablespoon olive oil
1 small onion, chopped
½ bell pepper, diced
3 cups sliced mushrooms (about ¾ pound)
3 or 4 leaves of bok choy (about 2 cups chopped)
2 tablespoons finely chopped parsley
2 teaspoons poultry seasoning
1 teaspoon salt, divided

¼ teaspoon black pepper
2 cups unsweetened fortified soy milk or rice milk
½ teaspoon onion powder
¼ teaspoon garlic powder
½ teaspoon salt
3 tablespoons rice flour
¼ cup potato flour
½ cup Corn Butter (page 201) or 3 tablespoons nonhydrogenated margarine
1 pound firm tofu, crumbled

Cook macaroni in boiling water until just tender, about 8 minutes. Drain and rinse, then set aside.

Heat olive oil in a large skillet and cook onion over high heat until soft, stirring occasionally, about 5 minutes.

Add bell pepper, mushrooms, bok choy, parsley, poultry seasoning, ½ teaspoon salt, and black pepper. Cover and cook until mushrooms are soft and bok choy is just tender, about 5 minutes.

Combine milk, onion powder, garlic powder, ½ teaspoon salt, rice flour, potato flour, and Corn Butter or margarine in a blender. Blend on high speed until mixture is thick and smooth.

Add to vegetables, along with crumbled tofu and cooked pasta. Stir to mix, then cook over medium-low heat, stirring frequently, until heated through, about 5 minutes.

> Per 1-cup serving: 273 calories; 12 g protein; 34 g carbohydrate;
> 11 g fat; 6 g fiber; 349 mg sodium; calories from protein: 17%;
> calories from carbohydrates: 49%; calories from fats: 34%

* * *

Fettucine with Broccoli and Pine Nuts
MAKES 8 1-CUP SERVINGS

This dish is perfect for a light supper. For a heartier meal, serve it with a bean soup and a crisp green salad.

8 ounces eggless fettucine	¼ teaspoon red pepper flakes or
1 tablespoon olive oil	pinch of cayenne
6 to 8 large garlic cloves, minced	1 28-ounce can crushed tomatoes
2 tablespoons pine nuts	1 bunch broccoli

Cook pasta according to package directions until tender. Pour off cooking water, then rinse and drain.

Heat oil in a large skillet and sauté garlic, pine nuts, and red pepper flakes or cayenne for 1 minute, stirring constantly.

Add tomatoes and simmer 7 minutes, stirring occasionally.

Break or cut broccoli into florets. Peel stems and slice into rounds. (You should have about 3 to 4 cups of broccoli.) Steam until crisp tender, about 5 minutes, then add to tomatoes.

Spread cooked pasta on a large platter and top with sauce. Serve immediately.

> Per 1-cup serving: 151 calories; 6 g protein; 26 g carbohydrate;
> 3 g fat; 4 g fiber; 218 mg sodium; calories from protein: 17%;
> alories from carbohydrates: 64%; calories from fats: 19%

* * *

Stuffed Eggplant
MAKES 6 SERVINGS

A man who hated eggplant (or thought he did) once declared this "the best meat I ever ate!"

3 small eggplants, 2½ to 3 inches in diameter
vegetable oil cooking spray
1 tablespoon olive oil
2 onions, chopped
4 garlic cloves, minced
2 bell peppers, seeded and diced
1½ cups chopped tomatoes (about 3 medium)
3 tablespoons chopped parsley
1 teaspoon basil
½ teaspoon salt
1 tablespoon nonhydrogenated margarine
¼ cup walnuts, chopped
¼ cup wheat germ

Preheat oven to 350°F.

Slice eggplants in half lengthwise and scoop out insides, leaving a ¼-inch thick shell. Place shells, cut sides down, in an oil-sprayed baking dish and bake until they just begin to soften, about 20 minutes. Set aside.

Coarsely chop eggplant flesh. Heat oil in a large nonstick skillet and add chopped eggplant, onions, garlic, and bell peppers. Cook over medium heat, stirring often, until eggplant begins to soften, about 10 minutes, adding a small amount of water if necessary to prevent sticking.

Add tomatoes, parsley, basil, and salt. Cook over medium heat until eggplant is tender when pierced with a fork, about 10 minutes. Divide among eggplant shells.

Melt margarine in a small pan, then stir in walnuts and wheat germ. Spread evenly over eggplant shells.

Arrange shells in one or two baking dishes. Bake, uncovered, until shells are completely tender when pierced with a fork, about 25 minutes.

Per ½ eggplant: 186 calories; 5 g protein; 26 g carbohydrate;
8 g fat; 7 g fiber; 209 mg sodium; calories from protein: 10%;
calories from carbohydrates: 52%; calories from fats: 38%

VEGETABLES
Red Potatoes with Black Bean Sauce
MAKES 4 SERVINGS

4 large red potatoes
1 15-ounce can black beans, drained
½ cup roasted red pepper
2 tablespoons lemon juice
2 tablespoons tahini (sesame butter)
½ teaspoon chili powder

¼ teaspoon cumin
¼ teaspoon coriander

¼ cup chopped fresh cilantro
2   green onions, finely chopped

Scrub potatoes and steam over boiling water until just tender when pierced with a fork, about 30 minutes.

While potatoes cook, puree black beans, roasted red pepper, lemon juice, tahini, chili powder, cumin, coriander, and cilantro in a food processor.

To serve, slit potatoes lengthwise. Press ends to open, then top with black bean sauce and chopped green onions.

Per 1-potato serving: 170 calories; 7 g protein; 31 g carbohydrate;
4 g fat; 8 g fiber; 805 mg sodium; calories from protein: 15%;
calories from carbohydrates: 67%; calories from fats: 18%

● ● ●

Curried Potatoes and Chickpeas
MAKES ABOUT 10 1-CUP SERVINGS

Serve this spicy dish with Brown Rice (page 176) and Cucumber Salad (page 191).

1   tablespoon olive oil
2   large onions, chopped
1   tablespoon whole cumin seeds
4   potatoes
1   15-ounce can crushed or ground tomatoes

1   15-ounce can garbanzo beans
1   teaspoon turmeric
1   teaspoon coriander
½ teaspoon ginger
¼ teaspoon cayenne
½ teaspoon salt

Heat oil in a large pot, then add onions and cumin seeds. Cook over high heat, stirring often, until onions are soft, about 5 minutes.

Scrub potatoes and cut into ½-inch cubes. Add to onions, along with tomatoes, garbanzo beans and their liquid, turmeric, coriander, ginger, cayenne, and salt. Bring to a slow simmer, then cover and cook, stirring occasionally, until potatoes are tender, about 25 minutes.

Per 1-cup serving: 202 calories; 7 g protein; 39 g carbohydrate;
3 g fat; 6 g fiber; 184 mg sodium; calories from protein: 14%;
calories from carbohydrates: 75%; calories from fats: 11%

● ● ●

Braised Collards or Kale
MAKES 3 1-CUP SERVINGS

Collard greens and kale are rich sources of calcium and beta-carotene as well as other minerals and vitamins. One of the tastiest—and easiest—

ways to prepare them is with a bit of soy sauce and plenty of garlic. Try to purchase young tender greens, as these have the best flavor and texture.

1 bunch collard greens or kale
   (6 to 8 cups chopped)
1 teaspoon olive oil
2 teaspoons reduced-sodium soy
   sauce

1 teaspoon balsamic vinegar
2 to 3 garlic cloves, minced

Wash greens, remove stems, then cut leaves into ½-inch wide strips.

Combine olive oil, soy sauce, vinegar, garlic, and ¼ cup water in a large pot or skillet. Cook over high heat about 30 seconds. Reduce heat to medium-high, add chopped greens, and toss to mix. Cover and cook, stir-ring often, until greens are tender, about 5 minutes.

Per 1-cup serving: 106 calories; 6 g protein; 18 g carbohydrate; 2 g fat; 6 g fiber; 132 mg sodium; calories from protein: 20%; calories from carbohydrates: 60%; calories from fats: 20%

● ● ●

Bok Choy

MAKES 3 1-CUP SERVINGS

Bok choy is another calcium-rich dark leafy green. The stems are crisp and tender, and can be sliced and cooked with the leaves.

2 bunches bok choy (about 6 cups
   chopped)
1 teaspoon olive oil

2 teaspoons reduced-sodium soy
   sauce
2 to 3 garlic cloves, minced
1 teaspoon balsamic vinegar

Wash bok choy, then slice leaves and stems into ½-inch strips.

Combine olive oil, soy sauce, garlic and ¼ cup water in a large pot or skillet. Cook over high heat about 30 seconds, then add bok choy and toss to mix.

Reduce heat to medium-high, then cover and cook, stirring often, until tender, about 5 minutes. Sprinkle with balsamic vinegar and toss to mix.

Per 1-cup serving: 60 calories; 4 g protein; 8 g carbohydrate; 2 g fat; 2 g fiber; 306 mg sodium; calories from protein: 23%; calories from carbohydrates: 41%; calories from fats: 36%

● ● ●

Broccoli with Sun-Dried Tomatoes
MAKES 4 1-CUP SERVINGS

The tangy flavor of sun-dried tomatoes is a perfect addition to steamed broccoli. Look for sun-dried tomatoes near the pickles and olives in your supermarket.

1 bunch broccoli	6 dried tomatoes in olive oil, drained

Rinse broccoli and cut into florets. Peel stems and slice into rounds. Steam over boiling water until just tender, 3 to 5 minutes.

While broccoli is cooking, cut tomatoes into small pieces and place in a serving dish. Add cooked broccoli to tomatoes, toss, and serve.

Per 1-cup serving: 40 calories; 4 g protein; 6 g carbohydrate; 0.8 g fat; 4 g fiber; 40 mg sodium; calories from protein: 29%; calories from carbohydrates: 55%; calories from fats: 16%

* * *

Zucchini Mexicana
MAKES 4 1-CUP SERVINGS

Serve as a vegetable side dish, or as a filling in warm corn tortillas.

2 teaspoons low-sodium soy sauce	1 cup corn kernels, fresh or frozen
1 onion, chopped	1 teaspoon cumin
3 garlic cloves, minced	1 teaspoon chili powder
3 cups diced zucchini	
1 red bell pepper, seeded and diced	

Heat soy sauce and ¼ cup water in a large skillet. Add onion and garlic. Cook over high heat, stirring often, until soft.

Add zucchini, bell pepper, corn, cumin, and chili powder. Reduce heat to medium and cook, stirring often, until zucchini is just tender, 3 to 5 minutes.

Per 1-cup serving: 80 calories; 4 g protein; 18 g carbohydrate; 0.6 g fat; 4 g fiber; 96 mg sodium; calories from protein: 16%; calories from carbohydrates: 77%; calories from fats: 7%

* * *

Italian-style Green Beans
MAKES 6 1-CUP SERVINGS

This colorful dish pleases the eye as well as the taste buds.

1 pound fresh green beans
1 tablespoon olive oil
2 cups chopped tomatoes, fresh or canned
2 large garlic cloves, minced

2 tablespoons chopped fresh basil or 1 teaspoon dried basil
salt and freshly ground pepper to taste

Trim ends off beans and cut or break into bite-size pieces. Steam until just tender, about 10 minutes, then set aside.

Heat oil in a large skillet, then add tomatoes and garlic. Simmer 10 minutes.

Add green beans and basil. Cook until beans are very tender, about 5 minutes, stirring occasionally. Add salt and pepper to taste.

Per 1-cup serving: 70 calories; 2 g protein; 10 g carbohydrate; 3 g fat; 4 g fiber; 120 mg sodium; calories from protein: 12%; calories from carbohydrates: 53%; calories from fats: 35%

● ● ●

Roasted Red Peppers
Roasted red peppers are delicious additions to salads, sauces, and soups. You can purchase water-packed roasted peppers in most grocery stores, or you can roast your own as described below.

1 (or more) large, firm red bell peppers

Wash pepper and place it over an open flame (such as a gas burner on the stove) or under the oven broiler. Turn pepper with tongs until skin is evenly charred on all sides.

Transfer to a bowl and cover with a plate. Let stand 15 minutes, then rub off charred skin. Cut pepper in half, saving any juice, and remove seeds. Use immediately or refrigerate or freeze for later use.

Per pepper: 20 calories; 0.6 g protein; 5 g carbohydrate; 0.1 g fat; 1 g fiber; 1 mg sodium; calories from protein: 11%; calories from carbohydrates: 83%; calories from fats: 6%

● ● ●

Roasted Garlic

Roasted garlic is a delicious appetizer or accompaniment to a meal. Serve it spread onto crusty French bread or mash it and add it to salad dressings. Store in a sealed container in the refrigerator for up to 2 weeks.

1 or more whole garlic heads

Preheat oven or toaster oven to 375°F.

Select heads of garlic with large cloves. Place entire bulb in a small baking dish and bake until cloves feel soft when pressed, about 35 minutes.

Microwave variation: Place 1 large head of garlic in microwave. Cook on high for 2 minutes, 10 seconds. Test for doneness with a fork.

Per bulb: 45 calories; 2 g protein; 10 g carbohydrate;
0.1 g fat; 0,6 g fiber; 5 mg sodium; calories from protein: 16%;
calories from carbohydrates: 82%; calories from fats: 3%

● ● ●

Wonderful Winter Squash
MAKES 8 1-CUP SERVINGS

Winter squash is available throughout the year in most places. If you've never tried a butternut, kabocha, or delicata you're in for a real treat. They can be steamed or baked, or prepared as described below.

1 winter squash   2 tablespoons maple syrup
1 tablespoon reduced-sodium soy
   sauce

Peel squash, cut in half and remove seeds. Cut squash into ½-inch cubes (you should have about 4 cups).

Put squash cubes in a large pot with ½ cup of water. Add soy sauce and maple syrup. Cover and simmer over medium heat, stirring occasionally, until squash is fork tender, 15 to 20 minutes.

Per 1-cup serving: 112 calories; 2 g protein; 28 g carbohydrate;
0.2 g fat; 6 g fiber; 136 mg sodium; calories from protein: 7%;
calories from carbohydrates: 91%; calories from fats: 2%

● ● ●

Cooking Potatoes, Sweet Potatoes, Yams and Winter Squash

Potatoes, sweet potatoes, and winter squash are traditionally baked, but steaming and microwaving are also an excellent methods for cooking these nutritious vegetables. In addition to being quick and easy, the vegetables stay moist and flavorful.

Steaming

To steam potatoes, yams, or sweet potatoes, simply scrub them (or peel them if you prefer) and arrange them on a steamer rack. Cook in a covered pot over simmering water until tender when pierced with a fork. This will take between 15 and 40 minutes, depending on their size. For quicker cooking, cut them into cubes or slices before steaming.

To steam winter squash, cut it in half and scoop out the seeds with a spoon. Cut it into wedges or other conveniently sized pieces and arrange on a steamer rack. Place in a pot, then cover and cook over medium heat until the squash is tender when pierced with a fork, between 15 and 30 minutes, depending on the size and freshness of the squash.

Microwave cooking

Russet Potatoes

2 medium potatoes

Pierce potato in several places with a fork. Place in microwave on rotating surface or turn midway during cooking. Microwave 7 to 8 minutes on high. Pierce with a fork to test for doneness. Crisp potato skins by placing in a toaster oven for a short time.

Sweet Potatoes or Yams

2 medium yams

Place yams in shallow covered casserole. Do not add water. Microwave 6 minutes on high, then turn yams over and microwave another 4 minutes. Test for doneness with a fork.

Butternut or Acorn Squash

1 squash

Cut squash in half and remove seeds. Place cut side down in a shallow dish. Do not add water. Microwave on high for 8 minutes. Turn squash right side up and cook another 6 minutes on high.

Orange-Glazed Sweet Potatoes
MAKES ABOUT 2 1-CUP SERVINGS

These golden sweet potatoes are a delicious addition to any meal.

2   medium sweet potatoes
3   tablespoons calcium-fortified
      orange juice concentrate
3   tablespoons maple syrup
$\frac{1}{4}$ teaspoon salt

Preheat oven to 350°F.

Peel sweet potatoes and cut into $\frac{1}{2}$-inch cubes (you should have about 2 cups). Place in a small covered baking dish.

Mix orange juice concentrate, maple syrup, and salt. Pour over sweet potatoes. Cover and bake until potatoes are tender when pierced with a fork, about 1 hour.

Per 1-cup serving: 238 calories; 2 g protein; 58 g carbohydrate;
0.2 g fat; 4 g fiber; 282 mg sodium; calories from protein: 4%;
calories from carbohydrates: 95%; calories from fats: 1%

● ● ●

Mashed Potatoes
MAKES ABOUT 10 $\frac{1}{2}$-CUP SERVINGS

Serve with Brown Gravy (page 202) and enjoy this traditional favorite to your heart's content!

4   russet potatoes, peeled and diced
1   cup unsweetened fortified soy
      milk or rice milk
$\frac{1}{4}$ teaspoon onion powder
$\frac{1}{4}$ teaspoon garlic powder
$\frac{1}{2}$ teaspoon salt
$1\frac{1}{2}$ tablespoons rice flour
2   tablespoons potato flour
$\frac{1}{2}$ cup Corn Butter (page 201) or
      1 tablespoon nonhydrogenated
      margarine

Put potatoes and 2 cups water in a saucepan. Simmer until potatoes are tender when pierced with a fork, about 10 minutes. Drain, reserving liquid. Mash potatoes.

Pour milk, onion powder, garlic powder, salt, rice flour, potato flour, and Corn Butter or margarine into a blender. Blend until completely smooth, about 1 minute. Add to mashed potatoes and stir to mix.

Per ½-cup serving: 85 calories; 2 g protein; 18 g carbohydrate; 1 g fat; 2 g fiber; 140 mg sodium; calories from protein: 11%; calories from carbohydrates: 81%; calories from fats: 8%

BREADS AND DESSERTS

Garlic Bread

MAKES ABOUT 20 SLICES

Roasted garlic makes a delicious, fat-free garlic bread. Choose heads with nice big cloves for easy peeling.

2 roasted garlic heads (see previous recipe)
1 to 2 teaspoons mixed Italian herbs

½ teaspoon salt
1 baguette or loaf of French bread, sliced

Preheat oven to 350°F.

Peel roasted cloves, or squeeze flesh from skin, and place in a bowl. Mash with a fork, then mix in Italian herbs and salt.

Spread on sliced bread. Wrap tightly in foil and bake for 20 minutes.

Per slice: 88 calories; 3 g protein; 17 g carbohydrate; 1 g fat; 1 g fiber; 229 mg sodium; calories from protein: 13%; calories from carbohydrates: 76%; calories from fats: 11%

● ● ●

Barley Scones

MAKES 12 SCONES

These tender scones are delicious plain or topped with fresh fruit. Barley flour is sold in natural food stores and some supermarkets.

¼ cup fortified vanilla soy milk or rice milk
2 tablespoons maple syrup
1 tablespoon canola oil
2 teaspoons vinegar
1 cup plus 3 tablespoons barley flour

¼ teaspoon baking soda
1 teaspoon baking powder
¼ teaspoon salt
3 tablespoons raisins
additional barley flour for dusting

Preheat oven to 350°F.

Mix milk, maple syrup, oil, and vinegar. Set aside.

Combine flour, baking soda, baking powder, salt, and raisins in a food processor. Blend until well mixed and raisins are chopped.

Add liquid ingredients and process until a ball of dough forms.

Transfer to a flat surface that has been dusted with barley flour. Flatten into a circle approximately 6 inches in diameter and ¾-inch thick. Use a sharp knife to score dough into 12 wedges (do not separate), then transfer to a baking sheet.

Bake for 30 minutes, until lightly browned.

Per scone: 117 calories; 3 g protein; 24 g carbohydrate;
1.5 g fat; 4 g fiber; 74 mg sodium; calories from protein: 9%;
calories from carbohydrates: 80%; calories from fats: 11%

● ● ●

Quick and Easy Brown Bread
MAKES 1 LOAF (ABOUT 20 SLICES)

This bread is made with healthful whole wheat and contains no added fat or oil. Serve it plain or with Pineapple Apricot Sauce (page 199).

1½ cups fortified soy milk or rice milk
2 tablespoons vinegar
3 cups whole wheat pastry flour
2 teaspoons baking soda
½ teaspoon salt
½ cup molasses
½ cup raisins

Preheat oven to 325°F.

Mix milk with vinegar and set aside.

In a large bowl, combine flour, baking soda, and salt. Stir to mix.

Add milk mixture and molasses. Stir to mix, then stir in raisins. Do not overmix.

Spread evenly in 5-by-9 inch nonstick or oil-sprayed loaf pan (pan should be about half full). Bake one hour.

Per slice: 100 calories; 3 g protein; 22 g carbohydrate;
1 g fat; 2 g fiber; 186 mg sodium; calories from protein: 12%;
calories from carbohydrates: 82%; calories from fats: 6%

● ● ●

Fresh Apple Muffins
MAKES 12 MUFFINS

These muffins make a satisfying breakfast or snack. Blackstrap molasses is a rich source of calcium and iron. It is not particularly sweet, however, thus the sugar in this recipe. If you choose to substitute regular unsul-

phured molasses, which is significantly sweeter, you can reduce the amount of sugar, or eliminate it altogether, depending on how sweet you like your muffins.

3 cups whole wheat pastry flour	1½ cups fortified soy milk or rice
½ cup sugar or other sweetener	milk
2 teaspoons baking soda	2 tablespoons cider vinegar
½ teaspoon salt	⅓ cup blackstrap molasses
2 cups finely chopped green apple	¾ cup raisins
(about 2 medium-large apples)	½ cup chopped walnuts (optional)

Preheat oven to 375°F.

Mix flour, sugar, baking soda, and salt. Set aside.

Put apples in a large mixing bowl and add milk, vinegar, and molasses. Add flour mixture and stir until just mixed, then stir in raisins and walnuts.

Spoon batter into oil-sprayed muffin cups, filling to just below tops.

Bake 30 to 35 minutes, until tops of muffins bounce back when lightly pressed.

Remove from oven and let stand about 5 minutes, then remove from pan and cool on a rack. Store in an airtight container.

Per muffin (with walnuts): 238 calories; 6 g protein; 48 g carbohydrate; 4 g fat; 5 g fiber; 310 mg sodium; calories from protein: 10%; calories from carbohydrates: 75%; calories from fats: 15%

Per muffin (without walnuts): 206 calories; 5 g protein; 47 g carbohydrate; 1 g fat; 5 g fiber; 310 mg sodium; calories from protein: 10%; calories from carbohydrates: 85%; calories from fats: 5%

● ● ●

Fresh Apricot Crumble
MAKES 9 SERVINGS

This is a perfect summer dessert when fresh apricots are abundant and flavorful.

4 cups coarsely chopped fresh	¼ cup sugar or other sweetener
apricots	¼ cup Corn Butter (page 201) or
2 tablespoons lemon juice	nonhydrogenated margarine
2 cups rolled oats	2 tablespoons water

Preheat oven to 350°F.

Toss chopped apricots with lemon juice and set aside.

Mix together rolled oats, sugar, and Corn Butter. Remove 1 cup and set aside. Add water to the remainder and mix until crumbly.

Pat oat mixture into an oil-sprayed 9-inch-square baking pan. Spread evenly with apricots and top with reserved crumb mixture. Bake for 35 to 40 minutes, until top crust is lightly browned.

Per serving: 143 calories; 4 g protein; 30 g carbohydrate; 2 g fat; 4 g fiber; 17 mg sodium; calories from protein: 12%; calories from carbohydrates: 78%; calories from fats: 10%

● ● ●

Butterscotch Pudding

MAKES 6 ½-CUP SERVINGS

This pudding gets its color from cooked yam and its flavor from Frontier Naturals Butterscotch Extract, which is sold in natural food stores.

2 cups fortified soy milk or rice milk
1 cup cooked, peeled yam
5 tablespoons maple syrup
2 tablespoons cornstarch
1 tablespoon potato flour
½ teaspoon Frontier Naturals butterscotch extract
¼ teaspoon salt

Combine milk, yam, and maple syrup in a blender and process until completely smooth. With the blender running, add cornstarch, potato flour, butterscotch extract, and salt.

Transfer to a saucepan and heat, stirring constantly, until mixture bubbles and thickens. Remove from heat and transfer to individual serving dishes if desired. Cool before serving.

Per ½-cup serving: 130 calories; 3 g protein; 26 g carbohydrate; 2 g fat; 2 g fiber; 133 mg sodium; calories from protein: 10%; calories from carbohydrates: 79%; calories from fats: 11%

● ● ●

Tapioca Pudding

MAKES 4 ½-CUP SERVINGS

Serve tapioca plain, or topped with Pineapple Apricot Sauce (page 199) or fresh fruit.

2 cups fortified soy milk or rice milk
¼ cup sugar
1 tablespoon potato flour
⅛ teaspoon salt
3 tablespoons instant tapioca
1 teaspoon vanilla extract

Stir together milk, sugar, potato flour, and salt in a saucepan. Add tapioca. Let stand 5 minutes, then bring to a boil over medium heat, stirring constantly.

Remove from heat and stir in vanilla. Transfer to individual serving dishes. Cool before serving.

Per ½-cup serving: 110 calories; 1.5 g protein; 25 g carbohydrate;
1 g fat; 1 g fiber; 68 mg sodium; calories from protein: 6%;
calories from carbohydrates: 88%; calories from fats: 6%

• • •

Cranberry Apple Crisp
MAKES 9 SERVINGS

Walnuts and rolled oats make a delicious topping for this colorful crisp.

3 tart green apples, peeled and cored	1½ cups quick-cooking rolled oats
3 tablespoons lemon juice	¾ cup walnuts, finely chopped
1 tablespoon sugar	⅓ cup maple syrup
1 teaspoon cinnamon	1 teaspoon vanilla extract
1 cup fresh or dried cranberries	¼ teaspoon salt

Preheat oven to 350°F.

Slice apples thinly and spread evenly in a 9-by-9-inch baking dish. Sprinkle with lemon juice, sugar, cinnamon, and cranberries.

Combine rolled oats, walnuts, maple syrup, vanilla, and salt in a bowl. Stir to mix, then spread evenly over apples.

Bake until apples are tender when pierced with a knife, about 35 minutes. Let stand 5 to 10 minutes before serving.

Per serving (⅑th of crisp): 197 calories; 4 g protein; 32 g carbohydrate;
7 g fat; 4 fiber; 61 mg sodium; calories from protein: 7%;
calories from carbohydrates: 61%; alories from fats: 32%

• • •

Fat-Free Banana Cake
MAKES 12 SERVINGS

This cake is delicious plain, or top it with Date Butter Frosting (recipe follows).

vegetable oil cooking spray	¾ cup maple syrup
3 cups whole wheat pastry flour	¾ cup fortified soy milk or rice milk
1 cup wheat germ	
2 teaspoons baking soda	2 teaspoons vanilla extract
¾ teaspoon salt	½ cup finely chopped dates or date pieces
6 ripe bananas	

Preheat oven to 350°F. Spray a 12-cup Bundt pan or 9-by-13-inch baking dish with cooking spray. Set aside.

Mix flour, wheat germ, baking soda, and salt.

Mash bananas in a large bowl. Mix in maple syrup, milk, and vanilla. Add flour mixture, then dates, and stir to mix.

Spread butter in prepared Bundt pan or baking dish. Bake for 55 minutes, until a toothpick inserted into the center comes out clean.

Per serving ($\frac{1}{12}$th of cake) without frosting: 234 calories; 7 g protein; 52 g carbohydrate; 2.5 g fat; 6 g fiber; 353 mg sodium; calories from protein: 10%; calories from carbohydrates: 82%; calories from fats: 8%

Per serving $\frac{1}{12}$th of cake) with frosting: 266 calories; 7 g protein; 58 g carbohydrate; 8 g fat; 3 g fiber; 301 mg sodium; calories from protein: 6%; calories from carbohydrates: 65%; calories from fats: 29%

• • •

Date Butter Frosting
MAKES ABOUT 1½ CUPS

This frosting stays soft and spreadable, so add a spoonful to each piece of cake as it is served.

1 cup fortified soy milk or rice milk
½ cup chopped pitted dates or date pieces
1 tablespoon cornstarch
½ teaspoon vanilla extract

½ teaspoon Frontier Naturals coconut extract
⅛ teaspoon salt
¼ cup Corn Butter (page 201) or nonhydrogenated margarine

Combine milk, dates, and cornstarch in a blender and process until smooth, 2 to 3 minutes on high speed.

Transfer to a saucepan and heat, stirring constantly, until mixture thickens and bubbles (it will have the consistency of pudding).

Remove from heat and stir in vanilla, coconut extract, and salt. When cool, mix in Corn Butter.

• • •

Pumpkin Raisin Cookies
MAKES 24 3-INCH COOKIES

These plump and moist cookies are perfect for an afternoon snack.

vegetable oil cooking spray
2 cups whole wheat pastry flour
½ cup sugar or other sweetener
2 teaspoons baking powder
½ teaspoon baking soda
½ teaspoon salt
½ teaspoon cinnamon

¼ teaspoon nutmeg
1 cup cooked or canned pumpkin
½ cup fortified soy milk or rice milk
½ cup raisins
½ cup chopped pecans or walnuts (optional)

Preheat oven to 350°F. Coat a baking sheet with cooking spray and set aside.

Mix flour, sugar, baking powder, baking soda, salt, cinnamon, and nutmeg together in a large bowl.

Add pumpkin, milk, raisins, and nuts. Mix completely.

Drop by tablespoonfuls onto prepared baking sheet. Bake 15 minutes, until bottoms are lightly browned. Remove from oven and let stand 2 minutes.

Carefully remove from baking sheet with a spatula and place on a rack to cool.

> Per cookie (with nuts): 79 calories; 2 g protein; 15 g carbohydrate;
> 2 g fat; 2 g fiber; 73 mg sodium; calories from protein: 9%;
> calories from carbohydrates: 72%; calories from fats: 19%

> Per cookie (without nuts): 63 calories; 2 g protein; 15 g carbohydrate;
> 0.2 g fat; 2 g fiber; 72 mg sodium; calories from protein: 10%;
> calories from carbohydrates: 88%; calories from fats: 2%

● ● ●

Tofu Cheesecake
MAKES 8 SERVINGS

This smooth and velvety "cheesecake," is delicious topped with fresh fruit or just the simple lemon glaze below. Agar flakes, which are made from seaweed, are used as a thickener. Look for them in natural food stores or Asian markets.

1 9-inch Fat-free Pie Crust (page 233) or baked crumb crust	2 teaspoons vanilla extract
2 tablespoons agar flakes	fresh fruit for topping (berries, kiwi fruit, mandarin orange segments, etc.) (optional)
⅔ cup fortified soy milk or rice milk	
½ cup sugar or other sweetener	*Lemon Glaze:*
½ teaspoon salt	⅓ cup sugar or other sweetener
1 pound reduced-fat firm tofu	1½ tablespoons cornstarch or arrowroot powder
4 tablespoons lemon juice	
2 teaspoons lemon zest	1½ tablespoons lemon juice
	½ teaspoon lemon zest

Combine agar flakes and milk in a saucepan and let stand 5 minutes. Stir in sugar and salt, then simmer over low heat, stirring frequently, for 5 minutes.

Pour into a blender and add tofu, lemon juice, lemon zest, and vanilla. Blend until completely smooth, 2 to 3 minutes. Spread evenly into crust. Chill 30 minutes then top with Lemon Glaze and fresh fruit if desired.

Stir sugar and cornstarch together in a small saucepan. Add lemon juice, zest, and ⅓ cup water. Whisk smooth.

Cook over medium heat, stirring constantly, until mixture is clear and thick. Spread evenly over cheesecake. Chill thoroughly before serving.

Per serving (⅛th of cake, with fruit): 233 calories;
7 g protein; 48 g carbohydrate; 3 g fat; 3 g fiber;
236 mg sodium; calories from protein: 11%;
calories from carbohydrates: 78%; calories from fats: 11%

* * *

Fat-Free Pie Crust
MAKES ONE 9-INCH CRUST

This crust is slightly sweet and chewy. It is much lower in fat and easier to prepare than traditional crumb crusts.

1   cup Grape-Nuts cereal   ¼ cup apple juice concentrate
                                        (undiluted)

Preheat oven to 350°F. Mix cereal and apple juice concentrate and pat into a 9-inch pie pan. Bake in preheated oven for 8 minutes. Cool before filling.

Per serving (⅛th of crust): 63 calories; 2 g protein; 15 g carbohydrate;
0.08 g fat; 1 g fiber; 97 mg sodium; calories from protein: 10%; calories
from carbohydrates: 89%; calories from fats: 1%

* * *

Fruit Gel
MAKES 8 ½-CUP SERVINGS

This is an all natural alternative to Jell-O! Agar powder and kudzu ("kood-zoo") are natural plant-based thickeners available in natural food stores.

1½ cups strawberries, fresh or   ½ teaspoon agar powder
      frozen   1   tablespoon kudzu powder
¾ cups apple juice concentrate   2   cups blueberries, fresh or frozen

Chop strawberries by hand or in a food processor.

Place in a pan with apple juice concentrate, ½ cup water, agar, and kudzu powder. Stir to mix.

Bring to a simmer and cook 3 minutes, stirring often. Remove from heat and chill completely.

Fold in blueberries and transfer to serving dishes.

Variations: Two cups of fresh or frozen blackberries or raspberries, or chopped peaches or mango may be substituted for the blueberries.

Per ½-cup serving: 77 calories; 0.5 g protein; 19 g carbohydrate;
0.2 g fat; 2 g fiber; 9 mg sodium; calories from protein: 2%;
calories from carbohydrates: 95%; calories from fats: 3%

BEVERAGES

Peach Smoothie
MAKES 3 TO 4 CUPS

This smoothie is reminiscent of fresh peach ice cream. You can freeze your own peaches when they are in season, or purchase frozen peaches at your supermarket.

2 peaches, sliced and frozen
1 to 2 cups fortified vanilla soy milk or rice milk

2 tablespoons undiluted apple juice concentrate

Combine all ingredients in a blender and process until smooth, 2 to 3 minutes. Serve immediately.

Per 1-cup serving: 96 calories; 4 g protein; 17 g carbohydrate;
2 g fat; 3 g fiber; 22 mg sodium; calories from protein: 15%;
calories from carbohydrates: 64%; calories from fats: 21%

● ● ●

Creamy Orange Freeze
MAKES 3 1-CUP SERVINGS

Serve this creamy orange drink with breakfast or as a mid-day cooler.

½ 12.3-ounce package Mori-Nu Lite Silken Tofu (firm)
1 ripe banana
½ cup calcium-fortified orange juice concentrate

1 cup fortified vanilla soy milk
2 tablespoons maple syrup
½ teaspoon vanilla
5 ice cubes

Combine all ingredients in a blender and process until completely smooth. Serve immediately.

Per 1-cup serving: 184 calories; 6 g protein; 39 g carbohydrate; 1 g fat;
1 g fiber; 38 mg sodium; calories from protein: 12%; calories from
carbohydrates: 81%; calories from fats: 7%

Glossary

Foods That May Be New to You

The majority of ingredients in the recipes are common and widely available in grocery stores. A few that may be unfamiliar are described below.

agar   a sea vegetable used as a thickener and gelling agent instead of gelatin, an animal by-product. Available in natural food stores and Asian markets. Also may be called "agar agar." Agar comes in several forms, including powder and flakes. The powder is the easiest to measure and the most concentrated form of agar. If a recipe calls for agar flakes and you are using powder, you will have to adjust the amount you use as follows: for each teaspoon of powder called for in the recipe, use approximately 1½ tablespoonfuls of flakes to substitute.

apple juice concentrate   frozen concentrate for making apple juice. May be used full strength as a sweetener.

arrowroot   a natural thickener that may be substituted for cornstarch.

baked tofu   tofu that has been marinated and baked until it is very firm and flavorful. Baked tofu is usually available in a variety of flavors. Sold in natural food stores and many supermarkets (check the deli and produce sections).

Bakkon yeast   a type of nutritional yeast with a smoky flavor. Also called "torula yeast." Sold in natural food stores.

balsamic vinegar   mellow-flavored wine vinegar that makes delicious salad dressings and marinades. Available in most food stores.

barley flour   can be used in baked goods in place of part or all of the wheat flour for a light, somewhat crumbly product. Available in natural food stores and many supermarkets.

Bob's Red Mill products   whole grain flours, multigrain cereal, and baking mixes. Contact the manufacturer to locate a source near you.

Bob's Red Mill Natural Foods, Inc.

5209 S.E. International Way

Milwaukee, OR 97222

800-553-2258

www.bobsredmill.com

Boca Burger   a low-fat vegetarian burger with a meaty taste and texture. Available in natural food stores, usually in the freezer case.

brown rice   an excellent source of protective soluble fiber as well as protein, vitamins, and minerals that are lost in milling white rice. Available in long-grain and short-grain varieties. Long-grain, which is light and fluffy, includes basmati, jasmine and other superbly flavorful varieties. Short-grain is more substantial and perfect for hearty dishes. Nutritionally there is very little difference between the two. Brown rice is sold in natural food stores and in many supermarkets.

bulgur   hard red winter wheat that has been cracked and toasted. Cooks quickly and has a delicious, nutty flavor. May be sold in supermarkets as "Ala."

carob powder   the roasted powder of the carob bean that can be used in place of chocolate in many recipes. Sold in natural food stores and some supermarkets.

couscous   although it looks like a grain, couscous is actually a very small pasta. Some natural food stores and supermarkets sell a whole wheat version. Look for it in the grain section.

date pieces   pitted, chopped dates that are coated with cornstarch to keep them from sticking together. They are sold in natural food stores and some supermarkets.

diced green chilies   refers to diced Anaheim chilies, which are mildly hot. These are available canned (Ortega is one brand) or fresh. When using fresh chilies, remove the skin by charring it under a broiler and rubbing it off once it has cooled.

Emes Jel   a natural gelling agent made from vegetable ingredients. May be combined with fruit juice to make a natural gelatin.

Fat-Free Nayonaise   a fat-free, cholesterol-free mayonnaise substitute that contains no dairy products or eggs. Sold in natural food stores and some supermarkets.

Fines Herbs   a herb blend that usually features equal parts of tarragon, parsley, and chives, and also may contain chervil. Look for it in the spice section.

garlic granules   another term for garlic powder.

Harvest Burger for Recipes   ready-to-use, ground beef substitute made from soy. Ideal for tacos, pasta sauces, and chili. Made by Green Giant (Pillsbury) and available in supermarket frozen food sections.

instant bean flakes   precooked black or pinto beans that can be quickly reconstituted with boiling water and used as a side dish, dip, sauce, or burrito filling. Fantastic Foods (707-778-7801) and Taste Adventure (Will-Pak Foods, 800-874-0883, www.tasteadventure.com) are two brands available in natural food stores and some supermarkets.

Italian Herbs   a commercially prepared mixture of Italian herbs: basil, oregano, thyme, marjoram, etc. Also may be called "Italian Seasoning." Look for it in the spice section of your market.

jicama ("hick-ama")   a crisp, slightly sweet root vegetable. Usually used raw in salads and with dips, but also may be added to stir-fries. Usually sold in the unrefrigerated area of the produce section.

kudzu ("kood-zoo")   a thickener made from the roots of the kudzu vine, which grows rampantly in the southeastern United States. It is used much like arrowroot or cornstarch and makes a creamy sauce or gel.

miso ("mee-so")   a salty fermented soybean paste used to flavor soup, sauces, and gravies. Available in light, medium, and dark varieties. The lighter-colored versions having the mildest flavor, while the dark are more robust. Sold in natural food stores and Asian markets.

nonhydrogenated margarine   margarine that does not contain hydrogenated oils. Hydrogenated oils raise blood cholesterol and can increase heart disease risk. Three brands of nonhydrogenated margarine are Earth Balance, Canoleo Soft Margarine, and Spectrum Spread.

nori ("nor-ee")   flat sheets of seaweed used for making sushi and nori rolls.

nutritional yeast   a good-tasting yeast that is richly endowed with nutrients, especially B vitamins. Certain nutritional yeasts, such as Red Star Vegetarian Support Formula Nutritional Yeast, are good sources of vitamin B_{12}. Check the label to be sure. Nutritional yeast may be added to foods for its flavor, sometimes described as "cheeselike," as well as for its nutritional value. Look for nutritional yeast in natural food stores.

Pacific Cream Flavored Sauce Base   a nondairy cream soup base made by Pacific Foods of Oregon and sold in natural food stores and many supermarkets.

potato flour   used as a thickener in sauces, puddings, and gravies. One common brand sold in natural food stores and many supermarkets is Bob's Red Mill.

prewashed salad mix, prewashed spinach   mixtures of lettuce, spinach, and other salad ingredients. Because they have been cleaned and dried, they store well and are easy to use. Several different mixes are available in the produce department of most food stores. "Spring mix" is particularly flavorful.

prune puree   may also be called "prune butter." Can be used in place of fat in baked goods. Commercial brands are WonderSlim and Lekvar. Prune baby food or pureed stewed prunes also may be used.

quinoa ("keen-wah")   a highly nutritious grain that cooks quickly and may be served as a side dish, pilaf, or salad. Sold in natural food stores.

red pepper flakes   dried, crushed chili peppers, available in the spice section or with the Mexican foods.

reduced-fat tofu   contains about a third of the fat of regular tofu. Three brands are Mori-Nu Lite, White Wave, and Tree of Life. Sold in natural food stores and supermarkets.

reduced-sodium soy sauce   also may be called "lite" soy sauce. Compare labels to find the brand with the lowest sodium content.

Rice Dream   see "rice milk."

rice flour   a thickener for sauces, puddings, and gravies. Choose white rice flour for the smoothest results. Bob's Red Mill is one common brand sold in natural food stores and many supermarkets.

rice milk   a beverage made from partially fermented rice that can be used in place of dairy milk on cereals and in most recipes. Available in natural food stores and some supermarkets.

roasted red peppers   red bell peppers that have been roasted over an open flame for a sweet, smoky flavor. Roast your own (see page 222) or purchase them already roasted, packed in water, in most grocery stores. Usually located near the pickles.

seasoned rice vinegar   a mild vinegar made from rice and seasoned with sugar and salt. Great for salad dressings and on cooked vegetables. Available in most grocery stores. Located with the vinegar or in the Asian foods section.

seitan ("say-tan")   also called "wheat meat," seitan is a high-protein, fat-free food with a meaty texture and flavor. Available in the deli case or freezer of natural food stores.

silken tofu   a smooth, delicate tofu that is excellent for sauces, cream soups, and dips. Often available in reduced-fat or "lite" versions. One popular brand, Mori-Nu, is widely available in convenient shelf-stable packaging—special packaging that may be stored without refrigeration for up to a year.

soba noodles   spaghetti-like pasta made with buckwheat flour. Has a delicious, distinctive flavor. Sold in natural food stores and in the Asian food section of some supermarkets.

sodium-free baking powder   made with potassium bicarbonate instead of sodium bicarbonate. Sold in natural food stores and some supermarkets. Featherweight is one brand.

soy milk   nondairy milk made from soybeans that can be used in recipes or as a beverage. May be sold fresh, powdered, or in convenient shelf-stable packaging. Choose calcium-fortified varieties. Available in natural food stores and supermarkets.

soy milk powder   can be used in smoothies, baked goods, or mixed with water for a beverage. Choose calcium-fortified varieties. Available in natural food stores and some supermarkets.

Spike a seasoning mixture of vegetables and herbs. Comes in a salt-free version, as well as the original version, which contains salt. Sold in natural food stores and many supermarkets.

spreadable fruit natural fruit preserves made of 100 percent fruit with no added sugar.

stone-ground mustard mustard containing whole mustard seeds. Often contains horseradish.

tahini ("ta-hee-nee") sesame seed butter. Comes in raw and toasted forms (either will work in the recipes in this book). Sold in natural food stores, ethnic grocery stores, and some supermarkets. Look for it near the peanut butter or with the natural or ethnic foods.

teff the world's smallest whole grain. Cooks quickly and has a rich, nutty flavor. Delicious as a breakfast cereal. Sold in natural food stores.

textured vegetable protein (TVP) meatlike ingredient made from defatted soy flour. Rehydrate with boiling water to add protein and meaty texture to sauces, chili, and stews. TVP is sold in natural food stores and in the bulk section of some supermarkets.

tofu a mild-flavored soy food that is adaptable to many different recipes. Texture varies greatly, from very smooth "silken" tofu to very dense "extra-firm" tofu. Flavor is best when it is fresh, so check freshness date on package.

torula yeast see "Bakkon yeast."

turbinado sugar also called "raw sugar" because it is less processed than white sugar.

unbleached flour white flour that has not been chemically whitened. Available in most grocery stores.

vegetable broth ready-to-use brands include Pacific Foods, Imagine Foods, and Swanson's. Other brands available in dry form as powder or cubes. Sold in natural food stores and many grocery stores.

wasabe ("wa-sah-bee") horseradish paste traditionally served with sushi. Sometimes sold fresh, but more commonly sold as a powder to be reconstituted. Look for it where Asian foods are sold.

whole wheat pastry flour milled from soft spring wheat. Has the nutritional benefits of whole wheat and produces lighter-textured baked goods than regular whole wheat flour. Available in natural food stores.

Yves Veggie Cuisine meatlike vegetarian products that are fat-free, including burgers, hot dogs, cold cuts, sausages, and Veggie Ground Round. Sold in natural food stores and many supermarkets.

Resources

Cookbooks

Bronfman, David and Rachelle. *Calciyum! Calcium-Rich, Dairy-Free Vegetarian Recipes.* Toronto, Ont., Canada: Bromedia, 1998.

Messina, Virginia, and Schumann, Kate. *The Convenient Vegetarian—Quick and Easy Meatless Cooking.* Hungry Minds, 1999.

Raymond, Jennifer. *Fat-Free and Easy: Great Meals in Minutes!* Book Publishing Company, 1997.

Stepaniak, Joanne. *Delicious Food for a Healthy Heart.* Summertown, Tenn.: Book Publishing Co., 1999.

Wasserman, Debra. *Simply Vegan: Quick, Vegetarian Meals.* Vegetarian Resource Group, 1999.

Nutrition

Barnard, Neal D. *Eat Right, Live Longer.* New York: Random House, 1995.

Barnard, Neal D. *Turn Off the Fat Genes.* New York: Harmony Books, 2001.

Davis, Brenda, and Melina, Vesanto. *Becoming Vegan.* Summertown, Tenn.: Book Publishing Company, 2000.

Lee, John R., M.D. *What Your Doctor May Not Tell You About Menopause.* New York: Warner Books, 1996

McDougall, John. *The McDougall Program for Women.* New York: Penguin Books, 1999.

Ornish, Dean M.D. *Eat More, Weigh Less.* New York: HarperCollins, 1993.

Physicians Committee for Responsible Medicine. WWW.PCRM.ORG

Traveling

Airplane travel.
    www.ivu.org/faq/travel.html
Directories on the Internet.
    www.vegdining.com and www.vegeats.com/restaurants
The Vegetarian Journal's Guide to Natural Foods Restaurants in the U.S. and Canada. Wayne, N.J.: Avery Publishing Group, 1998; updated every few years.

References

Chapter 1: Ageproofing from the Inside

Snow, K. K., and Seddon, J. M. "Do Age-Related Macular Degeneration and Cardiovascular Disease Share Common Antecedents?" *Ophthalmic Epidemiology* 6 (1999): 125–143.

Chapter 2: Making Sense of Nutrition

Abelow, B. J.; Holford, T. R.; and Insogna, K. L. "Cross-Cultural Association between Dietary Animal Protein and Hip Fracture: A Hypothesis." *Calcium Tissue International* 50 (1992): 14–18.

Baker, R. C.; Hogarty, S.; Poon, W.; et al. "Survival of Salmonella Typhimurium and Staphylococcus Aureus in Eggs Cooked by Different Methods." *Poultry Science* 62 (1983): 1211–1216.

Bush, A. L.; Pettingel, W. H.; Multhaup, G.; et al. "Rapid Induction of Alzheimer A-beta Amyloid Formation by Zinc." *Science* 265 (1994): 1464–1467.

Buzby, J. C., and Roberts, T. "ERS Estimates U.S. Foodborne Disease Costs." *Food Review* (USDA) (May-Aug 1995): 37.

Clyne, P. S., and Kulczycki, A. "Human Breast Milk Contains Bovine IgG. Relationship to Infant Colic?" *Pediatrics* 87 (1991): 439–444.

Feskanich, D.; Willett, W. C.; Stampfer, M. J.; and Colditz, G. A. "Milk, Dietary Calcium, and Bone Fractures in Women: A 12-Year Prospective Study." *American Journal of Public Health* 87 (1997): 992–997.

Chapter 3: Diet and the Menstrual Cycle

Barnard, N. D.; Scialli, A. R.; Hurlock, D.; and Bertron, P. "Diet and Sex-Hormone Binding Globulin, Dysmenorrhea, and Premenstrual Symptoms." *Obstetrics & Gynecology* 95 (2000): 245–250.

De Ridder, C. M.; Thijssen, J. H. H.; Van't Veer, P.; et al. "Dietary Habits, Sexual Maturation, and Plasma Hormones in Pubertal Girls: A Longitudinal Study." *American Journal of Clinical Nutrition* 54 (1991): 805–813.

Deutch, B. "Menstrual Pain in Danish Women Correlated with Low N-3

Polyunsaturated Fatty Acid Intake." *European Journal of Clinical Nutrition* 49 (1995): 508–516.

Kleijnen, J.; Ter Riet, G.; and Knipschild, P. "Vitamin B_6 on Premenstrual Symptomatology in Women with Premenstrual Tension Syndromes: A Double-Blind Crossover Study." *Infertility* 3 (1980): 155–165.

Thys-Jacobs, S.; Ceccarelli, S.; Bierman, A.; Weisman, H.; Cohen, M.; and Alvir, A. "Calcium Supplementation in Premenstrual Syndrome." *Journal of General Internal Medicine* 4 (1989): 183–189.

Chapter 4: Enhancing Fertility

Barr, S. I.; Janelle, K. C.; and Prior, J. C. "Vegetarian v. Nonvegetarian Diets, Dietary Restraint, and Subclinical Ovulatory Disturbances: Prospective 6-Mo Study." *American Journal of Clinical Nutrition* 60 (1994): 887–894.

Fairfield, K. "Annual Meeting of the Society for General Internal Medicine." *Obstetrics and Gynecology News* (June 15, 2000).

Grodstein, F.; Goldman, M. B.; Ryan, L.; and Cramer, D. W. "Relation of Female Infertility to Consumption of Caffeinated Beverages." *American Journal of Epidemiology* 37 (1993): 1353–1360.

Malter, M.; Schriever, G.; and Eilber, U. "Natural Killer Cells, Vitamins, and Other Blood Components of Vegetarian and Omnivorous Men." *Nutrition and Cancer* 12 (1989): 271–278.

Traill, K. N.; Huber, L. A.; Wick, G.; and Jurgens, G. "Lipoprotein Interactions with T Cells: An Update." *Immunology Today* 11 (1990): 411–417.

Chapter 5: A Healthy, Drug-Free Menopause

Herrington, D. M. "The HERS Trial Results: Paradigms Lost? Heart and Estrogen/Progestin Replacement Study." *Annals of Internal Medicine* 131 (September 21, 1999): 463–466.

Hulley, S.; Grady, D.; Bush, T.; et al. "Randomized Trial of Estrogen plus Progestin for Secondary Prevention of Coronary Heart Disease in Post-menopausal Women." *Journal of the American Medical Association* 280 (1998): 605–613.

Chapter 6: The Keys to Easy Weight Loss

Dayton, S.; Hashimoto, S.; Dixon, W.; and Pearce, M. L. "Composition of Lipids in Human Serum and Adipose Tissue during Prolonged Feeding of a Diet High in Unsaturated Fat." *Journal of Lipid Research* 76 (1996): 103–111.

Drenowski, A. "Taste Preferences and Food Intake." *Annual Review of Nutrition* 17 (1997): 237–253.

Lucchina, L. A.; Bartoshuk, L. M.; Duffy, V. B.; Marks, L. E.; and Ferris, A. M. "6-N-Propylthiouracil." *Chemical Senses* 20 (1995): 735.

Ludwig, D. S.; Majzoub, J. A.; Al-Zahrani, A.; Dallal, G. E.; Blanco, I.; and Roberts, S. B. "High Glycemic Index Foods, Overeating, and Obesity." *Pediatrics* 103 (1999): 656.

Mattes, R. D. "Fat Preference and Adherence to a Reduced-Fat Diet." *American Journal of Clinical Nutrition* 57 (1993): 373–381.

Nicholson, A. S.; Sklar, M.; Barnard, N. D.; Gore, S.; Sullivan, R.; and Browning, S. "Toward Improved Management of NIDDM: A Randomized, Controlled, Pilot Intervention Using a Low-Fat, Vegetarian Diet." *Preventive Medicine* 29 (1999): 87–91.

Wadden, T. A.; Foster, G. D.; Letizia, K. A.; and Mullen, J. L. "Long-Term Effects of Dieting on Resting Metabolic Rate in Obese Outpatients." *Journal of the American Medical Association* 264 (1990): 707–711.

Chapter 7: Cancer Prevention

Armstrong, B., and Doll, R. "Environmental Factors and Cancer Incidence"; Lingeman, C. H. "Etiology of Cancer of The Human Ovary: A Review." *Journal of the National Cancer Institute* 53 (1974): 1603–1618.

Christiansen, C. F.; Wang, L.; Barton, M. B.; et al. "Predicting the Cumulative Risk of False-Positive Mammograms." *Journal of the National Cancer Institute* 92 (2000): 1657–1666.

Cramer, D. W.; Willett, W. C.; Bell, D. A.; et al. "Galactose Consumption and Metabolism in Relation to the Risk of Ovarian Cancer." *Lancet* 2 (1989): 66–71.

Elwood, J. M.; Cole, P.; Rothman, J.; and Kaplan, S. D. "Epidemiology of Endometrial Cancer." *Journal of the National Cancer Institute* 59 (1994): 1055–1060.

Risch, H. A.; Jain, M.; Marrett, I. D.; and Howe, G. R. "Dietary Fat Intake and Risk of Epithelial Ovarian Cancer." *Journal of the National Cancer Institute* 86 (1994):1409–1415.

Welch, H. G.; Schwartz, L. M.; and Woloshin, S. "Are Increasing 5-Year Survival Rates Evidence of Success against Cancer?" *Journal of the American Medical Association* 283 (2000): 2975–2978.

Willett, W. C.; Stampfer, M. J.; Colditz, F. A.; et al. "Moderate Alcohol Consumption and the Risk of Breast Cancer." *New England Journal of Medicine* 316 (1987): 1174–1180.

Wynder, E. L.; Escher, G. C.; and Mantel, N. "An Epidemiological Investigation of Cancer of the Endometrium." *Cancer* 19 (1996): 489–520.

Chapter 8: Protecting Your Heart

Barnard, N. D.; Scialli, A. R.; Bertron, P.; Hurlock, D.; Edmonds, K.; and Talev, L. "Effectiveness of a Low-Fat, Vegetarian Diet in Altering Serum Lipids in Healthy Premenopausal Women." *American Journal of Cardiology* 85 (2000): 969–972.

Belcher, J. D.; Balla, J.; Balla, G.; et al. "Vitamin E, LDL, and Endothelium: Brief Oral Vitamin Supplementation Prevents Oxidized LDL-Mediated Vascular Injury in Vitro." *Arteriosclerosis Thrombosis, and Vascular Biology* 13 (1993): 1779–1789.

Bordia, A. "Effect of Garlic on Blood Lipids in Patients with Coronary Heart Disease." *American Journal of Clinical Nutrition* 34 (1981): 2100–2103.

Gould, K. L.; Ornish, D.; Scherwitz, L.; et al. "Changes in Myocardial Perfusion Abnormalities by Positron Emission Tomography after Long-Term Intense Risk Factor Modification." *Journal of the American Medical Association* 274 (1995): 894–901.

Hu, F.; Stampfer, M.; Colditz, G.; et al. "Physical Activity and Risk of Stroke in Women." *Journal of the American Medical Association* 283 (2000): 2961–2967.

Hunninghake, D. B.; Stein, E. A.; and Dujovne, C. A. "The Efficacy of Intensive Dietary Therapy Alone or Combined with Lovastatin in Outpatients with Hypercholesterolemia." *New England Journal of Medicine* 328 (1993): 1213–1219.

Liu, S.; Manson, J. E.; Stampfer, M.; et al. "Whole Grain Consumption and Risk of Ischemic Stroke in Women." *Journal of the American Medical Association* 284 (2000): 1534–1540.

Messina, M., and Messina, V. *The Simple Soybean and Your Health*. N.Y.: Avery Publishing Group, 1994.

Ornish, D.; Brown, S. E.; Scherwitz, L. W.; et al. "Can Lifestyle Changes Reverse Coronary Heart Disease?" *Lancet* 336 (1990): 129–133.

Sabate, J.; Fraser, G. E.; Burke, K.; Knutsen, S. F.; Bennett, H.; and Lindsted, K. D. "Effects of Walnuts on Serum Lipid Levels and Blood Pressure in Normal Men." *New England Journal of Medicine* 328 (1993): 603–607.

Chapter 9: Using Foods to Fight Arthritis

Aoki, S.; Yoshikawa, K.; Yokoyama, T.; et al. "Role of Enteric Bacteria in the Pathogenesis of Rheumatoid Arthritis: Evidence for Antibodies to Enterobacterial Common Antigens in Rheumatoid Sera and Synovial Fluids." *Annals of Rheumatic Diseases* 55 (1996): 363–369.

Belch, J. J. F.; Ansell, D.; Madho, K. A. R.; O'Dowd, A.; and Sturrock, R. D. "Effects of Altering Dietary Essential Fatty Acids on Requirements for Non-Steroidal Anti-Inflammatory Drugs in Patients with Rheumatoid Arthritis: A Double Blind Placebo Controlled Study." *Annals of Rheumatic Diseases* 47 (1988): 96–104.

Carman, W. J.; Sowers, M. F.; Hawthorne, V. M.; and Weissfeld, L. A. "Obesity as a Risk Factor for Osteoarthritis of the Hand and Wrist: A Prospective Study." *American Journal of Epidemiology* 139 (1994): 119–129.

Cauley, J. A.; Kwoh, C. K.; Egeland, G.; et al. "Serum Sex Hormones and Severity of Osteoarthritis of the Hand." *Journal of Rheumatology* 20 (1993): 1170–1175.

Cleland, L. G.; Hill, C. L.; and James, M. J. "Diet and Arthritis." *Ballière's Clinical Rheumatology* 9 (1995): 771–785.

Dayton, S.; Hashimoto, S.; Dixon, W.; and Pearce, M. L. "Composition of Lipids in Human Serum and Adipose Tissue during Prolonged Feeding of a Diet High in Unsaturated Fat." *Journal of Lipid Research* 76 (1966): 103–111.

Field, C. J., and Clandinin, M. T. "Modulation of Adipose Tissue Fat Composition by Diet: A Review." *Nutrition Research* 4 (1984): 743–755.

Gibson, T.; Rodgers, A. V.; Simmonds, H. A.; Court-Brown, F.; Todd, E.; and Meilton, V. "A Controlled Study of Diet in Patients with Gout." *Annals of Rheumatic Diseases* 42 (1983): 123–127.

Hart, D. J., and Spector, T. D. "The Relationship of Obesity, Fat Distribution, and Osteoarthritis in Women in the General Population: The Chingford Study." *Journal of Rheumatology* 20 (1993): 331–335.

Hicklin, J. A.; McEwen, L. M.; and Morgan, J. E. "The Effect of Diet in Rheumatoid Arthritis." *Clinical Allergy* 10 (1980): 463.

Hochberg, M. C. "Epidemiologic Considerations in the Primary Prevention of Osteoarthritis." *Journal of Rheumatology* 18 (1991): 1438–1440.

Hunter, J. E. "N-3 Fatty Acids from Vegetable Oils." *American Journal of Clinical Nutrition* 51 (1990): 809–814.

Inman, R. D. "Antigens, the Gastrointestinal Tract, and Arthritis." *Rheumatic Diseases Clinics of North America* 17 (1991): 309–321.

Kjeldsen-Kragh, J.; Haugen, M.; Borchgrevink, C. F.; et al. "Controlled Trial of Fasting and One-Year Vegetarian Diet in Rheumatoid Arthritis." *Lancet* 338 (1991): 899–902.

Kjeldsen-Kragh, J.; Haugen, M.; Borchgrevink, C.F.; and Forre, O. "Vegetarian Diet for Patients with Rheumatoid Arthritis—Status: Two Years after Introduction of the Diet." *Clinical Rheumatology* 13 (1994): 475–482.

Leventhal, L. J.; Boyce, E. G.; and Zurier, R. B. "Treatment of Rheumatoid Arthritis with Gammalinolenic Acid." *Annals of Internal Medicine* 119 (1993): 867–873.

Mantzioris, E.; James, M. J.; Gibson, R. A.; and Cleland, L. G. "Dietary Substitution with an Alpha-Linolenic Acid-Rich Vegetable Oil Increases Eicosapentaenoic Acid Concentrations in Tissues." *American Journal of Clinical Nutrition* 59 (1994): 1304–1309.

Packer L. "Interactions among Antioxidants in Health and Disease: Vitamin E and Its Redox Cycle." *Proceedings of the Society for Experimental Biology and Medicine* 200 (1992): 271–276.

Panush, R. S.; Carter, R. L.; Katz, P.; Kowsari, B.; Longley, S.; and Finnie, S. "Diet Therapy for Rheumatoid Arthritis." *Arthritis and Rheumatism* 26 (1983): 462–471.

Phinney, S. D.; Odin, R. S.; Johnson, S. B.; and Holman, R. T. "Reduced Arachidonate in Serum Phospholipids and Cholesteryl Esters Associated with Vegetarian Diets in Humans." *American Journal of Clinical Nutrition* 51 (1990): 385–392.

Pullman-Moor, S.; Laposata, M.; Lem, D.; et al. "Alteration of the Cellular Fatty Acid Profile and the Production of Eicosanoids in Human Monocytes by Gamma Linolenic Acid." *Arthritis and Rheumatism* 33 (1990): 1526–1533.

Ratner, D.; Eshel, E.; and Vigder, K. "Juvenile Rheumatoid Arthritis and Milk Allergy." *Journal of the Royal Society of Medicine* 78 (1985): 410–413.

Schnitzer, T. J.; Posner, M.; and Lawrence, I. D. "High Strength Capsaicin Cream for Osteoarthritis Pain: Rapid Onset of Action and Improved

Efficacy with Twice Daily Dosing." *Journal of Clinical Rheumatology* 1 (1995): 268–273.

Skoldstam, L. "Fasting and Vegan Diet in Rheumatoid Arthritis." *Scandinavian Journal of Rheumatology* 15 (1986): 219–223.

Spector, T. D.; Hart, D. J.; Brown, P.; et al. "Frequency of Osteoarthritis in Hysterectomized Women." *Journal of Rheumatology* 18 (1991): 1877–1883.

Srivastava, K. C., and Mustafa, T. "Ginger (*Zingiber Officinale*) in Rheumatism and Musculoskeletal Disorders." *Medical Hypotheses* 39 (1992): 342–348.

Watson, C. P. N.; Evans, R. J.; and Watt, V. R. "Post-Herpetic Neuralgia and Topical Capsaicin." *Pain* 33 (1988): 333–340.

Williams, R. "Rheumatoid Arthritis and Food: A Case Study." *British Medical Journal* 283 (1981): 563.

Chapter 10: Keeping Bones Strong

Abelow, B. J.; Holford, T. R.; and Insogna, K. L. "Cross-Cultural Association between Dietary Animal Protein and Hip Fracture: A Hypothesis." *Calcified Tissue International* 50 (1992): 14–18.

Felson, D. T.; Zhang, M. T.; and Hannan, M. T. "The Effect of Postmenopausal Estrogen Therapy on Bone Density in Elderly Women." *New England Journal of Medicine* 329 (1993): 1141–1146.

Feskanich, D.; Willett, W. C.; Stampfer, M. J.; and Colditz, G. A. "Milk, Dietary Calcium, and Bone Fractures in Women: A 12-Year Prospective Study." *American Journal of Public Health* 87 (1997): 992–997.

Frassetto, L. A.; Todd, K. M.; Morris, R. C. Jr.; and Sebastian, A. "Worldwide Incidence of Hip Fracture in Elderly Women: Relation to Consumption of Animal and Vegetable Foods." *The Journals of Gerontology, Series A, Biological Sciences and Medical Sciences* 55 (2000): 585–592.

Hopper, J. L., and Seeman, E. "The Bone Density of Female Twins Discordant for Tobacco Use." *New England Journal of Medicine* 330 (1994): 387–392.

Lemann, J.; Pleuss, J. A.; and Gray, R. W. "Potassium Causes Calcium Retention in Healthy Adults." *Journal of Nutrition* 123 (1993): 1623–1626.

Lloyd, T.; Chinchilli, V. M.; Johnson-Rollings, N.; Kieselhorst, K.; Eggli, D. F.; and Marcus, R. "Adult Female Hipbone Density Reflects Teenage Sports-Exercise Patterns but Not Teenage Calcium Intake." *Pediatrics* 106 (2000): 40–44.

Massey, L. K., and Whiting, S. J. "Caffeine, Urinary Calcium, Calcium Metabolism, and Bone." *Journal of Nutrition* 123 (1993): 1611–1614.

Nicar, M. J., and Pak, C. Y. C. "Calcium Bioavailability from Calcium Carbonate and Calcium Citrate." *Journal of Clinical Endocrinology and Metabolism* 61 (1985): 391–393.

Nordin, B. E.; Need, A. G.; Morris, H. A.; and Horowitz, M. "The Nature and Significance of the Relationship between Urinary Sodium and Urinary Calcium in Women." *Journal of Nutrition* 123 (1993): 1615–1622.

Remer, T., and Manz, F. "Estimation of the Renal Net Acid Excretion by Adults Consuming Diets Containing Variable Amounts of Protein." *American Journal of Clinical Nutrition* 59 (1994): 1356–1361.

Chapter 11: Free Yourself from Headaches

Abraham, G. E., and Hargrove, J. T. "Effect of Vitamin B6 on Premenstrual Symptomatology in Women with Premenstrual Tension Syndromes: A Double-Blind Cross-Over Study." *Infertility* 3 (1980): 155–165.

Brush, M. G. "Vitamin B6 Treatment of Premenstrual Syndrome." in *Clinical and Physiological Applications of Vitamin B₆: Current Topics in Nutrition And Disease,* vol. 19, ed. J. E. Leklem and R. D. Reynolds. New York: Alan R. Liss, 1988.

Chaytor, J. P.; Crathorne, B.; and Saxby, M. J. "The Identification and Significance of 2-Phenylethylamine in Foods." *Journal of the Science of Food and Agriculture* 26 (1975): 593–598.

Egger, J.; Carter, C. M.; Wilson, J.; and Turner, M. W. "Is Migraine Food Allergy? A Double-Blind Controlled Trial of Oligoantigenic Diet Treatment." *Lancet* 2 (1983): 865–869.

Groenewegen, W. A., Knight; D. W.; and Heptinstall, S. "Progress in the Medicinal Chemistry of the Herb Feverfew." *Progress in Medical Chemistry* 29 (1992): 217–238.

Hanington, E. *Migraine.* London: Priory Press, 1974.

Johnson, E. S.; Kadam, N. P.; Hylands, D. M.; and Hylands, P. J. "Efficacy of Feverfew as Prophylactic Treatment of Migraine." *British Medical Journal* 291 (1985): 569–573.

Littlewood, J. T.; Gibb, C.; Glover, V.; Sandler, M.; Davies, P. T. G.; and Rose, F. C. "Red Wine as a Cause of Migraine." *Lancet* 1 (1988): 558–559.

Mansfield, L. E.; Vaughan, T. R.; Waller, S. F.; Haverly, R. W.; and Ting, S. "Food Allergy and Adult Migraine: Double-Blind and Mediator Confirmation of an Allergic Etiology." *Annals of Allergy* 55 (1985): 126–129.

Murphy, J. J.; Heptinstall, S.; and Mitchell, J. R. A. "Randomised Double-Blind Placebo-Controlled Trial of Feverfew in Migraine Prevention." *Lancet* 2 (1988): 189–192.

Vaughan, T. R. "The Role of Food in the Pathogenesis of Migraine Headache." *Clinical Review of Allergy* 12 (1994): 167–180.

Vaughan, T. R.; Mansfield, L. E.; Haverly, R. W.; Chamberlin, W. M.; and Waller, S.F. "The Value of Cutaneous for Food Allergy in the Diagnostic Evaluation of Migraine Headaches." *Annals of Allergy* 50 (1983): 363.

Wantke, F.; Gotz, M.; and Jarisch, R. "The Red Wine Provocation Test: Intolerance to Histamine as a Model for Food Intolerance." *Allergy Proceedings* 15 (1994): 27–32.

Weaver, K. "Migraine and Magnesium" (letter). *Perspectives in Biology and Medicine* 33 (1989): 150–151.

Chapter 12: Urinary Tract Health

Avorn, J.; Monane, M.; Gurwitz, J. H.; Glynn, R. J.; Choodnovskiy, I.; and Lipzitz, L. A. "Reduction of Bacteriuria and Pyuria after Ingestion of Cranberry Juice." *Journal of the American Medical Association* 271 (1994): 751–754.

Curhan, G. C.; Willett, W. C.; Rimm, E. B.; Spiegelman, D.; and Stampfer, M. J. "Prospective Study of Beverage Use and the Risk for Kidney Stones in Women." *Annals of Internal Medicine* 126 (1997): 497–504.

Curhan, G. C.; Willett, W. C.; Rimm, E. B.; and Stampfer, M. J. "A Prospective Study of Dietary Calcium and Other Nutrients and the Risk of Symptomatic Kidney Stones." *New England Journal of Medicine* 328 (1993): 833–838.

Curhan, G. C.; Willett, W. C.; Speizer, F. E.; Spiegelman, D.; and Stampfer, M. J. "Comparison of Dietary Calcium with Supplemental Calcium and Other Nutrients as Factors Affecting the Risk for Kidney Stones in Women." *Annals of Internal Medicine* 126 (1997): 497–504.

Smith, S. D.; Wheeler, M. A.; Foster, H. E. Jr.; and Weiss, R. M. "Improvement in Interstitial Cystitis Symptom Scores during Treatment with Oral L-Arginine." *Journal of Urology* 158 (1997): 703–708.

Index

Note: An Index of Recipe Titles can be found on pages ix–x.